USING EVIDENCE IN HEALTH AND SOCIAL CARE

Using Evidence in Health and Social Care

This book forms part of the core text for the Open University course K302 *Critical Practice in Health and Social Care* and it is related to other materials available to students, including three more published texts:

- Critical Practice in Health and Social Care (Book 1)
- Changing Practice in Health and Social Care (Reader 1)
- Evaluating Research in Health and Social Care (Reader 2).

If you are interested in studying this course, or related courses, please write to the Information Officer, School of Health and Social Welfare, The Open University, Walton Hall, Milton Keynes MK7 6AA, UK.

Details are also given on our Web page at http://www.open.ac.uk

Using Evidence in Health and Social Care

Edited by

Roger Gomm and Celia Davies
The Open University

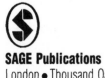

SAGE Publications
London ● Thousand Oaks ● New Delhi in association with The Open University

Sage Publications Ltd
6 Bonhill Street
London EC2A 4PU

SAGE Publications Inc
2455 Teller Road
Thousand Oaks, California 91320

SAGE Publications India Pvt Ltd
32, M-Block Market
Greater Kailash – I
New Delhi 110 048?tpb=6pt>

British Library Cataloguing in Publication data

A catalogue record for this book is available
from the British Library

ISBN 0 7619 6494 0 (hbk)
ISBN 0 7619 6495 9 (pbk)

Edited, designed and typeset by The Open University

Printed in the United Kingdom by T. J. International, Padstow, Cornwall

8720B/K302b2prelimsi1.1

Contents

Contributors

Meg Bond is an associate fellow in the Department of Continuing Education at the University of Warwick. She worked for many years as a practitioner, a lecturer and a researcher in the fields of vocational guidance, social work, and health care before becoming the co-ordinator of a community-based economic regeneration partnership project in the Midlands

Ann Brechin is a senior lecturer in the School of Health and Social Welfare at The Open University, where she has worked for 20 years. Her most recent books, edited with Open University colleagues, are *Critical Practice in Health and Social Care*, a companion volume to this one, and *Care Matters: Concepts, Practice and Research in Health and Social Care*, both published by Sage.

Celia Davies is Professor of Health Care at The Open University. She chaired the course team for K302 *Critical Practice in Health and Social Care*, this being one of the set texts. Her most recent book (with Abigail Beach) is *Interpreting Professional Self-Regulation: A History of the UKCC*, published by Routledge (forthcoming).

Maureen Eby is a senior lecturer in the School of Health and Social Welfare at The Open University. She is a nurse with a foot in both education and clinical nursing as she continues to practise in critical care at a local NHS acute hospital. Her writing was born out of her current research into whistleblowing and nursing negligence.

Roger Gomm is a lecturer in the School of Health and Social Welfare at The Open University, having previously worked in social work, social care and nurse training. He has been an author on a wide range of Open University courses, including *Educational Research Methods*, *An Ageing Society*, *Managing Roles and Relationships* and *Mental Health and Distress*. His interest in social science methodologies is reflected in *Case Study Research* (with Martin Hammersley) and *Evaluating Research in Health and Social Care* (edited with Gill Needham and Anne Bullman), a companion volume to this one and also published by Sage.

Elizabeth Hart is a senior lecturer at the University of Nottingham and Course Director of the Master of Science degree in Health Policy and Organisation. She is a social anthropologist whose research has included participant observation with domestic assistants and a study of recruitment and retention issues with nursing staff in two teaching hospitals. In 1995 she did a major action research study at a then District General Hospital, which formed the basis of an action research book with Meg Bond. Her most recent research is an evaluation of stroke services in the community.

Kelley Johnson is a senior lecturer and associate director of a research and consultancy unit on human services at Deakin University, Australia. She has firsthand experience of a wide range of research methods and has most recently worked in women's health, the sexual experience of young people and learning disability. Her latest published book is *Deinstitutionalising Women* (Cambridge University Press). She is now working (with R. Transtadottir) on a book called *Women and Intellectual Disability: Finding a Place in the World*.

Gill Needham is a librarian at The Open University and works closely with the School of Health and Social Welfare. She previously worked in the NHS in research and development roles, specialising in promoting evidence-based practice and public involvement in health care decision making. She has published work in both these areas. She is a managing partner of the NHS Centre for Health Information Quality, which was set up to promote the availability of high quality, evidence-based health information for the public.

Moyra Sidell is a senior lecturer in the School of Health and Social Welfare at The Open University. She was an author on the courses *Health and Wellbeing*, *Death and Dying* and *Promoting Health*. She has published in the fields of women's health and the health of older people and she is currently researching the care of dying older people in residential and nursing homes.

Acknowledgements

Grateful acknowledgement is made to the following sources for permission to reproduce material in this book.

Text

Chapter 2

Box 2: First published in the British Medical Journal. Cohen, G. *et al.* (1996) 'Can different patient satisfaction survey methods yield consistent results? Comparison of three surveys', *British Medical Journal*, 5 October, Vol. 313, No. 7061, pp. 841–4, reproduced by permission of the BMJ.

Chapter 5

Box 3: Lauri, S. and Sainio, D. (1998) 'Developing the nursing care of breast cancer patients: an action research approach', *Journal of Clinical Nursing*, Vol. 7, Blackwell Science Ltd; *Box 5:* Bond, E. *et al.* (1998) 'Knowing mothers: from practitioner research to self-help and organisational change', *Educational Action Research*, Vol. 6, No. 1, Triangle Journals Ltd.

Chapter 9

Pawson, R. and Tilley, N. (1997) *Realistic Evaluation*. Reprinted by permission of Sage Publications Ltd. © Sage Publications Ltd.

Chapter 11

Box 4: Williams, R. and Wright, J. (1998) 'Epidemiological issues in health needs assessment', *BMJ*, Vol. 316, p. 1382 and Payne, N. and Saul, C. (1997) 'Variations in use of cardiology services in a health authority ...', *BMJ*, Vol. 314, pp. 257–66 are reproduced by permission of the British Medical Journal.

Figures

Chapter 1

Figure 2: Reprinted by permission of Sage Publications Ltd from Crotty, M. (1998) 'Introduction: the research process', *The Foundations of Social Research*. © Michael Crotty, 1998. First published 1998 by Allen & Unwin Pty Ltd, Australia.

Chapter 5

Figure 1: Susman, G. I. and Evered, R. D. (1978) 'An assessment of the scientific merits of action research', *Administrative Science Quarterly*, Vol. 23. © 1978 by Cornell University.

Chapter 10

Figure 1: EuroQoL Group (1990) 'EQ-5D Questionnaire'. © EuroQoL Group. www.eurqol.org

Chapter 11

Figure 1: A Health Profile of Sheffield's Electoral Wards, Sheffield Health Authority (1994); *Figure 2:* Noble, M. and Smith, T. (1994) 'Children in need: using geographical information systems ...', *Children and Society*, Vol. 8, No. 4, National Children's Bureau Enterprises Ltd. Copyright John Wiley & Sons Limited. Reproduced with permission.

Tables

Chapter 2

Tables 1 and 2: First published in the British Medical Journal. Cohen, G. *et al.* (1996) 'Can different patient satisfaction survey methods yield consistent results? Comparison of three surveys', *British Medical Journal*, 5 October, Vol. 313, No. 7061, pp. 841–4, reproduced by permission of the BMJ; *Table 4:* Bosanquet, N. and Zarzecka, A. (1995) 'Attitudes to health services 1983 to 1993', in *Health Care UK 1994/95 – An Annual Review of Health Care Policy*, King's Fund Policy Institute.

Chapter 5

Table 1: Hart, E. and Bond, M. (1995) *Action Research for Health and Social Care: A Guide to Practice*, Open University Press.

Chapter 10

Tables 1 and 2: First published in the British Medical Journal. Shepperd, S. *et al.* (1998) 'Randomised controlled trial comparing hospital at home care with inpatient hospital care', *BMJ*, 13 June, Vol. 316, p. 1793, reproduced by permission of the BMJ; *Table 3:* Torrance, G. (1987) 'Utility approach to measuring health-related quality of life', *Journal of Chronic Diseases*, Vol. 40, No. 6 and Richardson, J. (1992) 'Cost–utility analyses in health care: present status and future issues', in Daly, J. *et al.* (eds) *Researching Health Care: Designs, Dilemmas, Disciplines*, Routledge/Taylor & Francis Ltd.

Every effort has been made to trace all the copyright owners, but if any have been inadvertently overlooked, the publishers will be pleased to make the necessary arrangements at the first opportunity.

Introduction

Government policy and professional guidance insist that professional practice should be 'evidence-based'. The pressure is on to justify both the choices made for particular clients and patients and the patterns of practice overall by reference to a body of evidence about efficiency and effectiveness. What does this mean for those who offer clinical services to patients in health settings and those who work with clients in social work and social care? Some gloomily see it as a matter of practice by protocol – ways of working that are more and more closely circumscribed with no room left for discretion, experience and judgement about the unique circumstances of the case. Others are excited by the prospect that custom and practice and the power of vested interests can be challenged by new insights and high quality research findings. Still others feel that the demands are impossible – 'How,' they ask, 'can anyone possibly keep up with the volume of research and decide what is relevant and what can be safely ignored?'

This book is addressed to all of these groups. It encourages them to ask 'What counts as evidence?' and to be active in considering the quality and relevance of research of different kinds to the practice in which they are engaged. It starts from the presumption, in the words of the title of Chapter 1, that there are different *ways of knowing*, that no one way is better in all circumstances and that the kinds of research done and the evidence produced will depend on the kinds of questions asked. This book also stresses *context-dependency* – however sound research is in its own terms, its relevance to a particular practical setting cannot be taken for granted. There is always a judgement to be made about the degree to which a new perspective or set of results can be transplanted from one setting to another. Thus, just as there is an active, professional assessment to be made with each client or patient encountered, so it is with the evidence on which future practice might be based. Good practice is a synthesis between professional experience, research evidence and the values and needs of the patient or client.

This book encourages the reader to 'unpick' the research that leads to the findings it reports and to bring to bear an understanding of the strengths and weaknesses of different research designs – what they reveal and what they leave hidden. This is very much the theme of Part 1. After a wide-ranging introductory chapter, Chapters 2–5 illustrate the mechanics of different types of research and indicate the different kinds of questions that need to be asked of each type. Chapter 10 does a similar job for economic analysis. This book also urges the reader to ask 'Is this research true for me?' In other words, does it translate into a particular setting? To answer this, it is necessary to know about the conditions of research production. Practitioners also sometimes need to know rather more than they do at present about the specific setting in which they seek to apply research. This is the theme of Part 2.

So, this is very much a practitioner's book. It is a book for people who want to read research and apply it in practice and not for people who want to do research themselves, for whom there are many excellent research manuals. It is also a book that assumes practitioners need to remain simultaneously interested and sceptical about the diversity of evidence from research, prepared both to challenge it and be challenged by it.

Many kinds of evidence

Much is heard today about the importance of the randomised controlled trial (RCT) as the 'gold standard' of research (Lawrence *et al.*, 1989). As Roger Gomm explains in Chapter 3, the logic of experimentation on which the RCT is based, the way in which its procedures enable variables to be controlled in order to avoid confounding is the closest we can get to certainty about cause and effect. The use of RCTs certainly increased in the 1990s and they have been applied to complex and multifaceted interventions. But not all evidence questions are causal questions and not all research problems are amenable to manipulation in the form of an experiment.

This line of thinking is explored most directly in Chapter 1. Ann Brechin and Moyra Siddell begin by pointing out that, in their daily work, practitioners in health and social care draw on different kinds of knowledge – empirical, theoretical and experiential – often moving seamlessly between them. Knowledge from observation, reasoning and experience, they argue, are not necessarily in competition but, instead, may feed into and enrich each other. Their remarks on the scientific method and what they call the 'positivist tradition', with its observational and experimental techniques, and the 'interpretivist tradition' recognise the strengths and weaknesses of both traditions and give an important context for the more detailed chapters that follow. Their vision is of a practitioner helped by the different research traditions discussed in this book, able to bring a critical eye and to search out studies using different methodologies, and to consider them in relation to both each other and the underlying concerns that informed them.

Chapters 2 and 3 exemplify Brechin and Siddell's positivist tradition. They illustrate the sceptical approach that the scientific method adopts to the possibility of ever knowing anything for certain. The question here, perhaps, is not 'How do I know a claim is true?' but rather 'How can I estimate the statistical chances of a claim being wrong?' In these two chapters Roger Gomm shows how survey and experimental research are predicated on the assumption that error is normal and on the belief that research needs to be designed to overcome the common human tendency to jump to conclusions that may well be wrong.

The chapter on survey methodology starts with a conundrum. How can two similar surveys of patient satisfaction in the NHS come up with different results? Are there real differences here, or are the results in some way an artefact of the design – attributable to differences in the way the studies were done? In engaging with these questions, Chapter 2 deals with the technical aspects of designing and conducting surveys and indicates the kinds of questions that need to be asked in appraising survey evidence. It also sets out five criteria for appraising the technical quality of research.

- *Reliability* – were the results free from the kinds of distortions that might arise from using methods inconsistently or using inconsistent methods?
- *Validity* – do the results accurately reflect what it is claimed they reflect?
- *Representativeness and generalisability* – are the findings true only of what was studied or would they be true more widely?
- *Fitness for purpose* – were the methods used appropriate for the purpose of the research?

Chapter 3 keeps these criteria in high profile. It is about experimental design and deals both with controlled experiments and with the experimental analysis of data collected from routine bureaucratic procedures or from surveys – so-called 'natural experiments'. Findings from RCTs are widely regarded as superior evidence about the effectiveness of health or social care interventions. Chapter 3 makes it clear that among controlled experiments the RCT is the most stringent design, with the strongest built-in safeguards against bias and against erroneously attributing outcomes to the effects of an intervention, rather than to other factors that have actually caused them. For this reason, the RCT can be seen as an ideal against which other experiments can be compared. However, there are circumstances where RCTs are not feasible. There are also circumstances where no controlled experiment is possible and researchers have to fall back on the 'natural experiment' to investigate matters of cause and effect. These alternatives are discussed in the chapter.

In health and social care, experiments have been the main source of producing sound knowledge about effective techniques of intervention, and surveys have been the main basis of knowledge about the causation of disease and social problems. In various combinations, the two approaches provide a basis for screening, risk assessment, needs assessment and performance indication and measurement. The four criteria – reliability, validity, and so on – can be applied across the range of techniques used here.

Where does this leave qualitative research? By comparison with quantitative research, it encompasses a much more diverse set of approaches. Qualitative research is often open-ended in that the researcher does not start with a question but allows questions to emerge from the data. Relationships between the researcher and the researched may be intense, and the studies may be long-term, broadly focused and conducted under naturalistic circumstances, which the researcher cannot control. Chapter 4 charts the move Kelley Johnson made from quantitative to qualitative research. While the study she describes uses participant observation, she ranges more widely. She gives glimpses of how grounded theory can refine concepts and develop and sometimes test theories in a limited way. In exploring the world view of a particular group, developing insights and concepts, and interpreting meanings, qualitative research comes into its own.

Chapter 4 can usefully be read in conjunction with a re-examination of Chapter 1, where the different assumptions of the interpretivist tradition are set out and compared with those that govern the positivist traditions exemplified by Chapters 2 and 3. Note that both approaches adhere to the importance of making research accountable to the reader through a detailed presentation of the way in which the results were obtained. The quantitative researcher sets store by reliability, giving details of design and measurements in such a way that someone else, using the same methods, might get the same results (replication). Qualitative researchers often manage this problem, as in Chapter 4, by giving a reflexive account – sharing their reflections on the research in progress with their readers. In a sense, this turns the procedure of the experimental tradition on its head – instead of seeking to remove or minimise researcher bias, they acknowledge and explore it, presenting it as part and parcel of the study (hence the biographical details and first-person style of the chapter).

Action research is the theme of Chapter 5. With its practical stress on problem solving and research done by or closely with practitioners with the express purpose of creating change, action research can often generate considerable local enthusiasm and commitment. Elizabeth Hart and Meg Bond trace some of the historical origins of the idea and its varying contemporary meanings. They define four kinds of action research and explore the distinctive features of each one. The notion that every approach has both strengths and weaknesses is addressed as they deal, on the one hand, with the way in which action research can give full rein to the complexities of problem definition and, on the other, with the charge that its findings are not generalisable. It is in the nature of action research that it collapses the temporal sequence of first finding things out, then subjecting the findings to peer review and then, if they survive the test, putting the findings into practice. In action research all this happens at the same time. Similarly, the division of labour between researchers, practitioners and research subjects may be abandoned, so that research becomes practice and practice research, which is welcomed in some quarters (Gibbons, 1994) and not in others.

There is the important question of whether all the research described in Chapters 2 to 5 can be assessed and evaluated according to a common set of criteria. Do the four criteria set out earlier always apply? Some authors have suggested that the list should be significantly modified or perhaps augmented to incorporate criteria such as acceptability to the researched, authenticity and trustworthiness (see, for example, Denzin and Lincoln, 1998). Kelley Johnson's discussion at the end of Chapter 4 expands on this point, urging that there may be diverse and irreconcilable views about the quality and usefulness of a particular piece of research. Hart and Bond in Chapter 5 conclude with a rather similar point when they refer to the salience of different kinds of evidence to different kinds of participants.

The place of ethics

Do we need reminding about the horrors of medical experimentation in the nineteenth century and of the German Third Reich? Do we need the rather more recent, but surely rare and extreme, examples of questionable research practice that Maureen Eby outlines at the start of Chapter 6? On the face of it, the answer is 'No'. There are now codes of practice and frameworks for the ethical review of research with human subjects and today's researchers are well aware of the need to obtain informed consent, to protect privacy and dignity, and to ensure that their interventions do no harm. Yet the position is not straightforward. It is by no means certain, as Chapter 6 points out, that participants always understand enough of the principles of randomisation and blinding underlying the experimental trial to realise what involvement in it will mean for them. As they do begin to grasp this, the personal risks both of the active intervention and of the placebo can seem shocking and unacceptable.

Nor is it only a matter of striving to put over the logic of the RCT and to secure informed consent to participation. Chapter 6 highlights ethical considerations that need to be explored for each type of research outlined in Part 1. It draws attention to power imbalances, the vulnerability of research subjects, and the threats to their privacy and dignity that need to be considered. It insists that conflicts of interest need to be recognised and that there is sometimes a difficult balance to be struck between the rigour of the research and respect for people. Users of research, as well as researchers themselves, need to consider the ethics of particular research designs; relevant ethical principles and frameworks to help with this are set out. Interestingly, the list of suggested questions for ethical review (Box 4 in Section 2) starts with the value of the research question being asked and the soundness of the research design to address it. If these questions cannot be answered satisfactorily, it is surely unethical to continue. A scientific appraisal and an ethical appraisal are not two different things – they are and should be closely bound together. This offers a way, perhaps, of expanding on the four criteria for technical quality set out earlier and of picking up on the invitation in Chapter 1 to use different lenses in viewing research evidence.

Dissemination, implementation and cross-mapping

For practitioners, the purpose of reading research is to find something that might be applied to their own practice. It is one thing to appraise a piece of research to estimate whether it is true in its own terms – whether it has *internal validity*. It is another thing to appraise research to estimate whether the findings might be true for other people in other places. This is the issue of *external validity* or generalisability – the transferability of research into practice.

Some of the problems of generalising derive from the research itself, from the nature of the samples used and the way the work is done. These are discussed in Part 1. But the problems of generalising also derive from the differences between the circumstances of the research and the circumstances in which its findings might be applied. The intervention in the experiment may have improved the condition of the majority of people involved. But gaining the same results in practice may not be possible unless practice features the same kinds of clients in the same kind of mix and the practitioner can do more or less the same as was done in the experiment. This is also true of the glimpses that qualitative writing gives of the world views of groups, institutions and practices, and of the findings produced through action research. The challenge of how to use research is reflected in the title of Part 2 – 'putting research into practice'. It forms the uniting theme for all the remaining chapters.

Viewed from the government departments who often fund research, the question of putting research into practice can frequently be seen as a matter of dissemination – making sure the right people get the right information about research results. The challenges then become informational – 'We must be sure that practitioners know about this research'. When that does not work, the issue gets translated into one of motivation or of cultural change – 'Why don't they take up the research in their own practice?'

In Chapter 7, Gill Needham reviews a range of so-called barriers to the implementation of evidence-based care. She argues for the importance of distinguishing clearly between the dissemination of information about effective practice and its implementation in practice and of working to improve both. The chapter charts the way in which efforts have been made in the NHS – through, for example, the development of clinical guidelines and the availability of systematic reviews – to package and distil relevant information about the latest evidence on best care for service-users. On their own, the chapter argues, these devices are not enough. Active implementation involving local ownership and adaptation are important. A local case study is used to suggest how information disseminated to users as well as practitioners can enable them to work together to change practice in the light of evidence and experience. Chapter 7 concludes, 'the practitioner needs to scrutinise research findings in the light of a detailed knowledge of local circumstances and the practice of their own organisation.'

This message is developed further by Roger Gomm in Chapters 8, 9 and 10, which are linked and follow from the observation that the outcomes of any piece of research are context-dependent. On these grounds, it is suggested that applying research to practice requires a *cross-mapping* exercise, comparing the circumstances under which the research was done with the circumstances under which some attempt will be made to emulate it. The more similar the two can be made, the more likely it is that research findings will travel.

Cross-mapping requires practitioners to know as much about what they are achieving in their practice as about the circumstances and techniques of the research. Chapter 8 addresses this by looking at the ways in which practice might be recorded, so that an informed decision can be made about whether there is a likelihood of something demonstrated in research being successful locally. In passing, the chapter also looks at the potential offered by information technology in this regard and at the difficulties some agencies have in demonstrating and recording their own effectiveness.

Chapter 9 carries the cross-mapping theme forward by examining the various ways in which contextual factors might vary between agencies and between an agency and a research location. Two multi-agency community crime-prevention schemes are used as case material. The kind of cross-mapping needed, the chapter implies, is not merely the 'tick-the-boxes' kind; it requires practitioners to have some kind of theory about how different factors influence each other, and what the critical ingredients for a successful intervention are (see Pawson and Tilley, 1997).

In Chapter 9 the issue of resources gets short shrift. This is because Chapter 10 is about economic analysis and variable resources are more conveniently dealt with there. The term 'economic analysis' implies an exclusive interest in money. However, as the chapter shows, important costs and benefits in economic analysis are not always monetary ones. Chapter 10 uses a case study of a cost-effectiveness analysis of a hospital at home scheme. As with many cost-effectiveness analyses, this one follows from a controlled experiment of the kind discussed in Chapter 3. This showed that ordinary in-patient care and hospital at home care were equally effective in promoting post-operative recovery, and almost equally effective in producing patient and carer satisfaction. Hence a decision between the two kinds of provision might be made on the grounds of cost. The chapter demonstrates the mechanics of this kind of analysis, and makes the important point that, of all kinds of quantitative research, cost-effectiveness analysis is the most context-sensitive of all. This is because the cost bases of different agencies vary considerably and the cost matrix can change dramatically over a short period of time. Sensitivity analysis, the economists' response to this problem, is illustrated. The reader is asked to regard any published cost–value analyses as useful models, but ones into which they should substitute costs drawn from their own agency.

The second part of Chapter 10 looks at QALYs – Quality-Adjusted Life Years – which are used in various kinds of economic analysis as a currency for judging the value of different outcomes. QALYs are put to practical use in two contexts. One is in many resource-allocation decisions and is controversial, although most of the controversy derives from the need to ration expenditure, rather than from the use of QALYs in doing so. The other context is assisting clients to make an informed choice between different treatments in the face of uncertain outcomes. At this point Chapter 10 relates back to remarks made in Chapter 3 about the way in which experimental research produces evidence about what is likely to happen to a group of people, but not about what is likely to happen to any one of them in particular. Chapter 10 uses the discussion of QALYs to illustrate the use of decision analysis to bridge the gap between evidence about outcomes for groups of people and decisions about individuals.

Chapter 11, the final chapter, again by Roger Gomm, shifts from decisions about individual clients to strategic decisions about the configuration of services. It is written around a major case study of a partnership of agencies putting together a bid for an award under the Single Regeneration Budget (SRB) scheme. This stands as an exemplar for bidding in terms of any 'challenge' funding and, to some extent, for any strategic planning process at local authority or health authority level. The question is 'How might evidence from research inform this planning?' The chapter deals with demographic models. These are important in themselves and because they form the basis for extrapolating from epidemiological research done elsewhere to predict the local pattern of diseases and social problems – a link here to Chapters 2 and 3. Chapter 11 pays particular attention to the use of deprivation indicators in determining the share-out of national health and welfare resources, in predicting local epidemiological patterns and in setting appropriate base-line standards for judging agency performance. The case study also features a survey designed to elicit majority local opinion about options for the SRB bid and gives an opportunity to revisit some of the remarks about surveys in Chapter 2. After this chapter, the book is rounded off with a brief appendix, which gives the reader signposts to finding the kinds of research discussed and indicates some of the sources of help, particularly electronic library help, that are increasingly available in this fast-changing world.

Different claims, different questions

Overall, this book shows that choosing a research method always involves trade-offs. The biggest of these is between methods that are well designed for investigating cause and effect (Chapters 2 and 3) and those that are better designed for investigating the ways in which people experience their lives (Chapter 4). Another trade-off relates to an iron law of research: that, for the same quantity of resources, a researcher can learn either a lot about a few people or a little about many; that the researcher has to choose between depth and breadth, meaningfulness and representativeness.

Similarly, a controlled experiment can achieve a high degree of control over variables and, hence, a high degree of internal validity, but the circumstances thus created may be so unusual and artificial that the results will not be generalisable to practice situations. However, a survey which studies things that happen under natural circumstances may have a high level of generalisability from sample to population but, because it exercises little control over variables, it may be unable to determine what caused what. Usually, the greatest strength of a method in one respect is also its greatest weakness in another. The practitioner–user of research always needs to ask 'How does this kind of research work?' and 'Has this author made it work properly?' Taken together, the chapters in this book are designed to help the reader use such questions in day-to-day practice.

It would be odd, to say the least, if a book encouraging its readers to question the origins of evidence and the context of production of evidence did not make clear its own context and origins. This volume of essays was written for the Open University third-level course K302 *Critical Practice in Health and Social Care*. The aim of the course is to encourage constructive reflection on practice and greater understanding of the context of contemporary health and social care, and to promote a shared awareness across disciplines and occupational groups of the changing contexts of practice and the growing need to work across boundaries. A substantial part of the course is devoted to research and evidence and to developing the knowledge and skills to deal with research evidence and to consider its applicability in different settings; this book forms the basic text to aid this learning. Its companion text, *Evaluating Research in Health and Social Care* (Gomm *et al.*, 2000), gives more details on methodological issues than here. It also reproduces a series of exemplar articles from across the health and social care field, showing how reading them can be enhanced by using resources and checklists found in the book and elsewhere in the course.

Open University authors gather more debts than is usual during the production of an academic text. We want to thank members of the K302 course team, critical readers and developmental testers who commented on earlier drafts of the chapters as the course was being developed, and the editors and administrative and clerical staff, all of whom helped to bring this book to fruition.

References

Denzin, N. K. and Lincoln, Y. S. (1998) (eds) *Strategies of Qualitative Inquiry*, London, Sage.

Gibbons, M. (1994) *The New Production of Knowledge: The Dynamics of Science and Research in Contemporary Societies*, London, Sage.

Gomm, R., Needham, G. and Bullman, A. (eds) (2000) *Evaluating Research in Health and Social Care*, London, Sage in association with The Open University (K302 Reader 2).

Lawrence, R., Friedman, G. and DeFriese, G. (1989) *Guide to Clinical Preventative Services: An Assessment of the Effectiveness of 169 Interventions. Report of the US Preventative Services Task Force*, Maryland, Williams and Wilkins.

Pawson, R. and Tilley, N. (1997) *Realistic Evaluation*, London, Sage.

Part 1
Evidence for Practice

Chapter 1
Ways of knowing

Ann Brechin and Moyra Sidell

Introduction

'Good morning,' said Deep Thought ...

'Er ... Good morning, O Deep Thought,' said Loonquawl nervously, 'do you have ... er, that is ...'

'An answer for you?' interrupted Deep Thought majestically. 'Yes, I have.'

The two men shivered with expectancy. Their waiting had not been in vain.

'There really is one?' breathed Phouchg.

'There really is one,' confirmed Deep Thought.

'To Everything? To the great Question of Life, the Universe and Everything?'

'Yes.'

Both of the men had been trained for this moment, their lives had been a preparation for it, they had been selected at birth as those who would witness the answer, but even so they found themselves gasping and squirming like excited children.

'And you're ready to give it to us?' urged Loonquawl.

'I am.'

'Now?'

'Now,' said Deep Thought.

They both licked their dry lips.

'Though I don't think,' added Deep Thought, 'that you're going to like it.'

'Doesn't matter!' said Phouchg. 'We must know it! Now!'

'Now?' inquired Deep Thought.

'Yes! Now ...'

'Alright,' said the computer and settled into silence again. The two men fidgeted. The tension was unbearable.

'You're really not going to like it,' observed Deep Thought.

'Tell us!'

'Alright,' said Deep Thought. 'The Answer to the Great Question ...'

'Yes ... !'

'Of Life, the Universe and Everything ...,' said Deep Thought.

'Yes ... !'

'Is ...,' said Deep Thought, and paused.

'Yes ... !'

'Is ...'

'Yes ... !!! ...?'

'Forty-two,' said Deep Thought, with infinite majesty and calm.

(Adams, 1979, pp. 134–5)

Health and social care workers are quite reasonably expected to know what they are doing. They are paid to practise on the basis that what they say or do will be well judged, appropriate and based on an informed appraisal of alternatives. At the very least they should know what to do better than the next person and the above answer, from *The Hitch Hiker's Guide to the Galaxy*, would not help them much. In a sense this whole book explores how far practitioners can, or do, know what they are doing and this first chapter sets the scene by reflecting on that question a little. How might people come to know? And how would anyone else know that they know? What is it, indeed, to know – anything? And not least, as the above quotation reminds us, what kinds of answers to what kinds of questions might it be useful to know?

Practitioners are likely to draw on different 'ways of knowing', moving in and out of them seamlessly or engaging in them simultaneously, often without being aware of the process. Such 'formal' and 'informal' knowing (see, for example, Thompson, 1995) may include the following.

- *Empirical knowing*: where a practitioner may know how to respond on the basis of the available research evidence. This is probably the most explicit form of knowing.

- *Theoretical knowing*: where a practitioner may recognise different theoretical frameworks for thinking about a problem, providing alternative ways of approaching it. This is public knowledge but it is often used intuitively and informally.

- *Experiential knowing*: where craft knowledge builds up over years of experience and involves a kind of tacit knowledge. This can be particularly hard to make explicit.

On the whole, knowledge about anything is accepted as such when there is widely shared public agreement about it. So most people now know that the Earth is round, whereas once they knew with equal certainty that it was flat. Nurses once knew it was important to keep people in bed, whereas now, in similar circumstances, they know how essential it is to get people up and about. Where knowledge is challenged or not widely agreed, we tend to talk in terms of beliefs. Religious beliefs, for example in God or Allah, are often cited as the classic sticking point, where individuals may claim to 'know' but, given the discrepancies, both cannot be exactly right. The 'widely shared agreement' thus tends to be contextual – knowledge exists in a context of time, space and culture and reflects the dominant belief system at that point. It reflects, in a sense, what is believed to be true on current evidence – or, more accurately, on the perceptions and interpretations of evidence that is seen as relevant by those who are in a position to influence wider beliefs.

The reason why it is important to think explicitly about how we come to 'know' things, and on what basis such knowing is accepted, is that such knowledge affects what we do. This involves the purposes that may drive research. In this chapter we suggest three overarching and overlapping concerns, portrayed in Figure 1 as three lenses through which the world may be viewed. The research enterprise will look different and be approached differently depending on which lens, or which combination of lenses, acts as a view-finder. Thinking in very simple terms like this about the interests that may motivate researchers can sometimes be helpful. You and others may give any number of reasons for wanting to know things, but the three lenses here seem to encapsulate most possible motives quite successfully, bearing, as they do, more than a passing resemblance to Habermas' (1972) conceptualisation of three fundamental human interests. One or more lenses may be operating at any one time, reflecting the personal and political concerns behind the very human and universal wish to know and to develop 'knowing'.

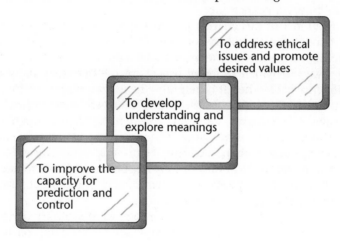

To address ethical issues and promote desired values

To develop understanding and explore meanings

To improve the capacity for prediction and control

Figure 1   **Three lenses: overarching and overlapping concerns driving a desire to know**

Whichever lens we look through, 'knowing' provides the basis on which we act in relation to other people and on which we intervene in events. The more our actions are seen as appropriate, the sounder the knowledge base will be perceived to be. And the more such predictions are questioned or contested on the basis of unhelpful or unforeseen outcomes, or because they fail to make sense to other people or in other situations, the more the knowledge base will be open to challenge. Practitioners are in a position of intervening in people's very lives, assessing and predicting the outcomes of various options. And they are working in a complex territory where certainty is always out of reach. It is little wonder there is so much concern to address and shore up the evidence base for practice. At least, the argument goes, practitioners should know the basis on which they think they know what they are doing!

This chapter looks at ways of knowing as they are enshrined and understood in different research traditions. Of the three ways of knowing listed above, the first – empirical knowing – lends itself most obviously to the call for evidence-based practice. But, as this book will make clear, there are many forms of knowledge and not all of them are associated with empirical traditions. Human behaviour has always been influenced by processes of seeking to know better – to understand, to predict, to become more skilled at interacting with the environment and with other people. Formalised research traditions, as they have evolved, are manifestations of a much larger and longer-lasting search reaching back through the centuries. Philosophers, seers, prophets and politicians, not to mention ordinary people, have long sought to build a working knowledge of life as we know it. Their concerns, like ours today, were with prediction and control, understanding and meaning, and ethics and values. For good or for ill, they wanted to engage more effectively with other people and with the world around them and they struggled to do so, rather like today's practitioners, through a combination of empirical observation, theoretical reasoning and experience.

Section 1 of this chapter provides some initial mapping of the relevant methodological territory for research in the health and social care field, highlighting some of the most visible landmarks, and suggesting some of the ways in which different aspects of methodology hang together and influence each other. It is helpful to have a starting point for exploring the rather complex interrelationships between such things as different purposes, paradigms, theories, research traditions, methodologies and methods. At the same time, though, there are clearly many ways of drawing such a map, defining terms and accounting for a range of different features that may or may not be brought into focus. This book as a whole necessarily reflects similar choices about what to feature rather than attempting to cover everything.

Sections 2 and 3 expand on the somewhat arbitrary divisions between the broad churches of positivist and interpretivist approaches. These can be seen as primarily, but not exclusively, reflecting concerns with the lens of prediction and control on the one hand and that of understanding and meaning on the other. Section 4 brings the third lens to the forefront by focusing on the interrelationships between power and perspectives and the different ways and purposes of knowing.

1   The methodological field

One of the challenges of presenting a neat map of 'the methodological field' is that it is hard to say where the boundaries lie and what the nature of interrelationships may be. Almost any attempt will oversimplify. One

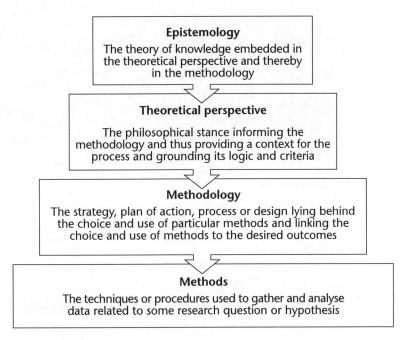

Figure 2   **Four elements that inform one another** (Source: based on Crotty, 1998, pp. 3–4)

succinct map of how different levels of any research process connect with or even nest into each other is offered by Crotty (1998) (see Figure 2).

The boundaries between the different elements are not absolute or discrete, but it can be helpful to recognise that the choice of method is not just a straightforward and rational question about which is most appropriate. Rather, quite complex moral, philosophical and political belief systems, as well as perhaps practical considerations, will profoundly affect the nature of the research.

The approach taken in this chapter will not differ fundamentally from Crotty's framework but, rather, it will present some of the implied territories and some of the relationships between them in a different way. Figure 2 presents an account of 'elements informing one another' (Crotty, 1998, p. 3) – epistemology informing theoretical perspective, in turn informing methodology and finally the methods chosen. The process is seen as linear and one-way and has the great advantage of seeming tidy and logical. It is important also, however, to acknowledge the rather messy and confusing way in which such influences, frameworks and approaches can interact – in several directions. Take theoretical perspectives for example, the second layer on Crotty's model. The mapping in Figure 3 (overleaf) suggests what these might include: a range of relevant discipline areas along with some related theories, models or frameworks of thinking that may be influential. These are shown as representing bio-psycho-socio-cultural fields of influence, borrowing from Cooper *et al.*'s

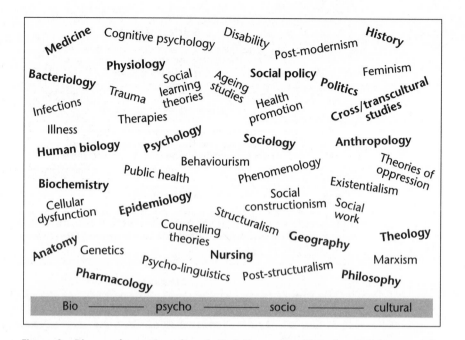

Figure 3   Bio-psycho-socio-cultural discipline areas, theories and frameworks

(1996) concept of a bio-psycho-social model of health and stretching it one important notch further.

Such a heaving mass of creative and interrelating theory and practice as this picture represents can be seen as the field from which research ideas, methodologies and methods emerge (following the arrows down on Figure 2). But the influences are not just one-way. New ideas will continually be feeding back, not just from research results but from the very processes of engaging in research design and execution. Wider influences will also impinge from beyond the confines of formal research as other ways of knowing jostle for position and influence to challenge and create new perspectives. Epistemologies and paradigm shifts, as Crotty indicates (Figure 2), will influence, underpin and constrain much of this theorising. But again it is not just a one-way and linear process. Those same theories of knowledge and paradigms of thinking will themselves be challenged and stretched by new ideas, theorising and feedback that may emerge from the pragmatic processes and discoveries at the end of the research chain and beyond.

It would equally be possible to argue for bio-psycho-socio-cultural *methodologies* as the underpinning fields of influence from which strategies and theories emerge – or *epistemologies*/paradigms (as Crotty does by implication). A case could even be made for research *methods* as being the field from which other ideas emerge. After all, new ideas and thinking often evolve directly from the challenges of developing new methods and being alert to new discoveries and observations. The development of feminist methods (for example, Maynard, 1994) serves to illustrate how the challenge of devising new methods had a strong influence as part of the development of the thinking as a whole. This is to argue, in essence, that methods are not just a technical matter.

However, we shall stay with the notion of the discipline and theoretical frameworks as forming the methodological field within which the research occurs. The mapping in Figure 4 (overleaf) shows the three other frameworks of influence embedded in this theoretical field:

- the broad epistemological (theories of knowledge) or paradigm frameworks, shown in terms of positivist or interpretivist positions
- the methodological or research strategy frameworks, shown as 'hypothesis testing', 'addressing research questions' or 'hermeneutic enquiry'
- methods tending to fall to one end or the other of the positivist or interpretivist ends of the scale or, in some cases, somewhere in between.

The two-way influences between epistemology/paradigm and methodology/research strategies are shown. (These terms are not exactly interchangeable, but we have opted to use both as a reminder of the rather imprecise and overlapping nature of some of these notions.) The diagram also shows two-way influences between methodology/research strategies and methods. Finally, arrows also indicate the links between methods and epistemologies and all of them both seep into and feed from the theoretical medium in which they are grounded.

Most of the terms used in Figure 4 are discussed further in the rest of this chapter and elsewhere in the book. Particular examples of research strategies and methods, for example, are covered in more detail in Chapters 2–5. Figure 4 is not intended to be exhaustive in its coverage, but it forms a map to which other concepts could be added. If we could present it in three dimensions, we might add the lenses from Figure 1 as an extra element, hovering over the methodological field, each affecting how it might be seen. Through the 'prediction and control' lens perhaps the left-hand positivist side might be most clearly in focus; through the 'understandings and meanings' lens perhaps the view would be better to the right where interpretivism holds sway; and perhaps the 'ethics and values' lens would offer a wide sweep over the centre ground extending far to both sides. The power and capacity to influence and to understand, as well as the ethical considerations involved, however, can and do depend on all kinds of knowledge. There are no clear lines of demarcation across this complex territory.

2   Positivist frameworks

This section focuses on traditions that seek to develop knowledge about what is talked of as the 'natural world'. This connects with some of the very powerful and dominant discourses reflected in the 'scientific method'

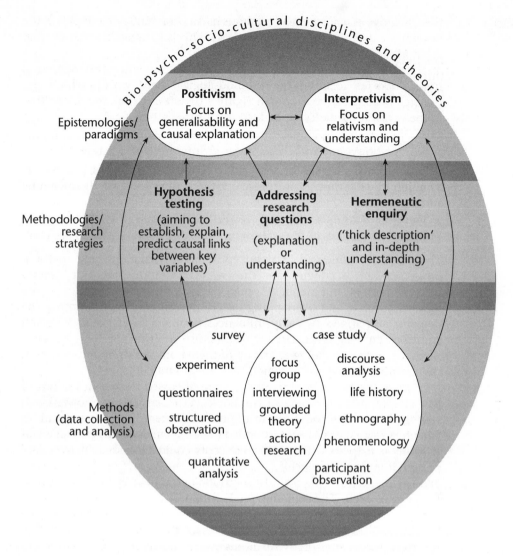

Figure 4 **The methodological field**

(see, for example, Usher, 1997; Hughes, 1990; Crotty, 1998; or Black, 1993, all of which contain summary accounts of this tradition). This has been the preferred route forward in most of the Western scientific world for at least the last century. The 'scientific method' offers powerful and important ways of thinking about knowledge, not just because it has been dominant but also because it offers very rigorous and explicit ways of challenging and checking claims to certain kinds of knowledge. It offers strategies for trying to ensure that claims to 'know better' than another, or 'better' than before, can be put to the test.

Objectivity, positivism and the real world

Positivism assumes the natural world can be apprehended directly through the perceptual and mental processes available to us. The scientific method is the research method that has evolved to understand, describe, explain and control the natural world, using observational and experimental methods to shore up our uncertain mental capacity by building in checks against bias. It aims to enable us to 'know better' by achieving greater objectivity. Objectivity becomes a counterbalance to the unreliability and variability of personal, or subjective, impressions and accounts by requiring that the basis of any observations should be essentially public and replicable.

The positivist tradition argues that knowledge about the world can only be gained through accumulating facts that have been discovered through controlled, replicable and objective observation or experiment. Laws and theories can then be derived from those accumulated facts. Such laws and theories will only become established if they have the power to predict accurately in new situations. In other words, they must be capable of generalisation to other settings and circumstances. Box 1 summarises the basic premises of the positivist tradition.

Box 1: A positivist paradigm

1 Some features of the world exist independently of knowers, i.e. they are 'objective'. This objective world includes events and phenomena that are lawful and orderly. Through systematic observation and correctly applied scientific methods, in particular by being 'objective', this lawfulness can be discovered – to explain, predict and control events and phenomena.

2 A distinction can be made between the 'subjective' knower and the 'objective' world. A clear distinction is also made between facts and values, the former seen as belonging to the objective world, the latter to the subjective knower. Subjectivity (the concerns, values and particularity of the researcher) is recognised as likely to interfere with perceptions and interpretations. Research methods try to mitigate against such effects.

3 Although subjectivity may affect our capacity to come to 'know' the natural world as it really is, there is an expectation that objective knowledge can be attained. Under reasonably controlled circumstances, different people would rationally be expected to reach the same conclusions, based on observation enhanced by experiment and measurement. This partly depends on a further assumption that a reasonably clear correspondence can be attempted between the world we experience and the language we use to represent and discuss it.

(Source: adapted from Usher, 1997)

Popper (1959, 1963) challenged the absolute certainty claimed by the extreme positivist position and argued for a scientific method based on a continual process of checking on claims to knowledge. He argued that, in order to find a universally applicable theory, a hypothesis must be not so much verifiable as falsifiable. Verification, he claimed, could never be achieved whereas falsification is possible. Popper's classic example was 'all swans are white'. The truth of this statement is not verifiable once and for all because, however many white swans are observed, there is always the possibility of finding a non-white swan. But as soon as a black swan is observed, it becomes possible to state categorically that not all swans are white. Thus the scientific method proposes that the best knowledge to be had about the world is that which has been subjected to a rigorous attempt to disprove it, and so far has survived such tests. Science never produces certain knowledge, only knowledge about which it is reasonable to be less uncertain.

What scientific method does bring about, though, is a culture of healthy scepticism: a readiness to doubt claims and assumptions about the 'rightness' of any particular theory or intervention; and a drive to apply rigorous methods to test whether a prediction is accurate, or whether something works, in what circumstances and with what degree of success. The measure of certainty with which anything can be said to be known depends then on the probability of there being any other explanation, such as that it might have happened by chance.

Being objective about people

Laws and theories about people, their health and well-being, their illnesses and distress, their patterns of behaviour and relationships are particularly hard to achieve. Nevertheless, many of the huge strides in modern medicine in particular (although also in many other fields) owe their knowledge base to the rigorous scepticism of the scientific method. Rather like in a court of law, the burden of proof rests with the scientist and the case for the prosecution. 'It was the blood-letting and leeches what did it, m'lud. Look, you can see how healthy she is now.' The defence argues the 'null hypothesis', i.e. that there is not a causal link. 'She might have recovered just as well, or even better, on her own. Here are a hundred others, untreated, m'lud, of whom only five are actually dead; and a hundred who were treated, ten of whom are dead and fifteen who suffer acute fevers after his doctoring.' In such a case, the intervention failed to demonstrate its helpfulness in bringing about a cure (although leeches are now thought to have particular beneficial effects on some wounds). It is, however, almost impossible to prove beyond doubt that an idea is right. Ultimately, the proof will rest on the balance of probabilities.

The chances of recovery with or without blood-letting can be calculated. The more cases there are, the more confidence can be placed in any findings. At the end of the day, that kind of knowing rests on the statistical probability of quantifiable outcomes. We can know that this or that intervention probably does or does not have this or that effect because the chances of this particular outcome occurring by chance are statistically very remote.

The knowledge base for practice in health and social care depends on a range of ways of knowing. Such knowledge varies in the extent to which it is, or can be, tested by scientific method, although other methods may be equally rigorous in different ways (as we shall see in Chapter 4). In social care, for example, judging whether interventions are helpful includes making some decisions about the meanings attached to outcomes, how those are valued and from whose point of view. Locking up young offenders or taking an abused child into foster care may be right from some points of view and wrong from others and the actual experience may vary substantially from one young person to the next. The short or long-term outcomes may also be different and be seen differently. In addition, many other factors, such as educational or employment opportunities and available housing, may profoundly affect what happens. In nursing, too, and in any therapeutic intervention, the process and the outcome will vary, in terms of health or rehabilitation, with a host of factors.

None of this means, however, that applying scientific method is not appropriate; only that it will be challenging to do so and possibly limited in the range of variables that can be addressed. Increasingly, practice is required to be evidence-based and that usually means based on research which uses at least the principles of scientific method, through experiments or surveys with statistical analysis of results indicating levels of significance. So, although it may be hard to do, and although it may provide information about only one kind of 'knowing' – a 'knowing' that assumes a real world of real people out there, available to be measured and judged as long as we can find the right methods for measuring and judging reliably – it is nevertheless important. It is hard to deny the reasonableness of a requirement to prove that what is being done in the name of professional help probably has some useful impact and that it is more useful than either doing nothing or doing something different.

3 Interpretivism

Different subject matter – different methods?

People form part of the natural world and, as such, can quite appropriately be explored and understood using means developed to research that world. A great deal has been, and continues to be, learned using the methods of the natural sciences. Such research underpins much of what the various human services offer by way of support and intervention. It is also arguable, however, that people are uniquely different from the rest of the natural world in being conscious and purposive creatures, whose past, present and projected future social, cultural and, to a considerable extent, environmental contexts are created by themselves. Dilthey (1833–1911), for example, argued that 'nature and culture were inherently different and required different methods of study' (quoted in Hughes, 1990, p. 90; see also Dilthey, 1976).

Figure 4 shows hermeneutic enquiry as the principal methodological strand, or 'different method of study', within the interpretivist paradigm. Hermeneutics was the term originally applied to the deciphering of ancient manuscripts – often biblical ones. The challenge was not just a linguistic one – to decode the lettering and the language – but also essentially a matter of contextual and historical interpretation. To grasp the meanings of the texts, or other evidence, involved trying to see into the minds and lived experiences of the people of those times and circumstances.

Hermeneutic enquiry in social sciences research today involves essentially the same process: the continuing attempt to access meanings by a thorough perusal of such evidence as can be made directly available and an understanding, as far as possible, of the context in which they (the observable actions) have occurred. It involves not so much a translation as an interpretation that will be influenced inevitably by the perspectives, experiences and expectations of the interpreter.

> Whenever something is interpreted as something, the interpretation will be founded essentially upon fore-having, fore-sight and fore-conception. An interpretation is never a presuppositionless apprehending of something presented to us.
>
> (Heidegger, 1962, p. 191)

Instead of seeing personal perceptions, interpretations or judgements as potential forms of contamination, interest shifts to how, as human beings, researchers do actually make sense of what they research. Hans-Georg Gadamer, a hermeneuticist, believes that knowledge emerges as we learn to question continually our prejudices and amend our assumptions (Warnke, 1987). This becomes a dialectic process as we move back and forth between our pre-assumptions and what is being revealed. This 'hermeneutic circle' can be seen as the basis of some phenomenological methodology (Finlay, 1999). Much of this thinking can be traced back to the work of the German philosopher Immanuel Kant (1724–1804), and his idea that history, culture and even the self are created by human beings and that these creations have to be understood by different methods from those appropriate to understanding nature.

Kant made a key distinction between the phenomenological world, the world as it appears to us, and the 'noumenal' world, the world as it is. He maintained that both were real but that each was different in its knowability. Other philosophers, including Max Weber (1864–1920) in particular, argued that such a distinction was misleading. Just as we cannot know directly about 'lived experiences' – particularly those of other people (except in so far as we can describe and interpret them through our senses or any other tools of measurement we can devise) – so we cannot know the outer world directly either. The essential tasks and assumptions of research and enquiry are thus the same. Weber's concern was to develop methodologies appropriate to understanding social phenomena, including causal relationships, which met the same standards of objectivity and rigour as the natural sciences (Weber, 1962).

These arguments may all seem rather esoteric in relation to what actually happens in health and social care. Whether there is a real social world in the same way as there is a real natural world, and whether we need the same or different tools and methodologies to research and understand them, seems a far cry from the world of dealing in the here and now with pain or unhappiness. But actually, it is not. As soon as you start to wonder about the pain or unhappiness – how to understand their (often multiple) causes; how best to help – you are drawn straight back into some of these fundamental issues. How can we know about the other person's experience? In what sense is the experience a reality that can be grasped and understood? Even our own experience of pain or unhappiness is ephemeral and will be felt and interpreted differently at different times and in different circumstances. Language itself, as a potential tool to help us access such understandings, is constituted according to many social constructionist thinkers (for example, Harré, 1986; Gergen and Gergen, 1991; von Glaserfeld, 1991; Shotter and Gergen, 1989; Potter, 1996) through an ongoing process of creating meanings through shared perceptions, understandings and actions.

What comes into the frame, then, is not so much a drive to establish knowledge (in the sense of known and predictable facts about causal relationships) as a concern to know and understand more about the nature and experience of living and being in relationship with the world and other people. In this sense, the nature of knowing itself becomes contested territory.

Different questions – different emphasis?

Interpretivist research tends to fall into the broad category known as qualitative research. Often, although not always, qualitative research asks questions that tend to elicit descriptive accounts. It is like asking 'What is going on here?' Goffman (1968) asked it about asylums; Menzies (1960) asked it about hospital routines; Bowlby (1988) asked it about children's attachments to primary carers. In such situations the kind of answer that is going to be useful is one offering a new way of seeing and understanding what is happening. Research stemming from this kind of thinking and questioning tends to be seen as qualitative rather than quantitative research because there is less likelihood of being able to count anything or make any numerically based judgements about the findings.

A simple illustration of what this can mean in practice is given in Box 2. It concerns understanding what was happening when people with a potentially life-threatening condition were failing to adhere to a treatment regime that could save their lives. By exploring the complexities of the respondents' daily lives in detail, this question could be addressed.

Box 2: Research on adherence to a drug regime

This research was done in Australia by a GP whose practice deals almost exclusively with people with HIV and AIDS. Although the recent discovery of HAART therapy has literally given people with AIDS a new lease of life, there is a worrying trend in those prescribed this life-saving medication of non-adherence to the treatment regimes. Surveys of people with AIDS have identified side-effects as the only statistically significant problem. From her impressions from her clinical practice, this GP was not convinced by these findings and did in-depth interviewing with all her patients who were prescribed the drugs.

She found that her patients' difficulties were seemingly trivial but very understandable. The HAART drug regimes have to be extremely rigid. Patients must take regular doses at very particular times in relation to meals. Missing a dose is dangerous and can render the treatment useless as well as create tolerance to the drugs. The lifestyle of this particular population is not regular and many patients talked of how they might spontaneously stay with friends over a weekend and not have their somewhat cumbersome medication with them.

Others whose lives were more regular or who were in work found it difficult taking their medication in public. Having to take medication with lunch could be difficult because they would have to explain what they were taking. Many did not want their colleagues to know that they had AIDS because of the stigma associated with it. Through the discovery of these and other similar intricate obstacles to adhering to their treatment regime, this GP was able to work with her patients and get them to identify their potential difficulties and work out strategies to counter them. She had managed to raise the adherence rate of her patients to well over 90%, which is much higher than other rates.

(Source: based on Workman, 1998)

The research involved going beyond the observed behaviour of the individuals, namely non-adherence to the drug regime, to find out something about their experiences – or at least their accounts of their experiences. However, it is worth making two points. First, 'knowing' that the treatment worked was an important starting point and one that was arrived at by other means, most likely through a fairly strict randomised controlled trial (see Chapter 3 for an explanation of this particular form of experimental research design). Secondly, the usefulness of the GP's analysis of the difficulties is not a foregone conclusion. No matter how much detail she unearthed, the question of its relevance remained uncertain. It may have felt relevant to her and to her patients, but that may have been to do with the kinds of questions she asked and what they thought she wanted to hear. They may have offered what seemed to both parties to be a plausible explanation for their risky non-adherence. Arguably, this is all that matters. In Box 2, however, additional value is placed on the GP's interpretation in that the strategies then developed enabled her to achieve a 90% adherence ('much higher than other rates'). To pursue this further, we might still need to ask some more quantitative questions: for example, was this rate significantly higher than other rates; did the strategies transfer in terms of impact to new patients; or was there an effect stemming simply from her interest in and involvement with the patients which made them much more inclined to try to comply? For example, feeling understood may have made them more positive in many ways, including their inclination to make the effort to protect their health.

   This turns out to be not an account of competing strategies but a nice illustration of how different ways of knowing, or different kinds of questions, can interconnect, feed into and enrich each other. As with all research, it involves a continual process of asking questions and checking out the answers. For example, a conversation with the GP at the time might have gone as follows: 'What have you noticed?' – a worrying level of non-compliance; 'Isn't it because of the side-effects?' – I'm not convinced; 'What else might it be?' – I don't know, maybe a life-style thing, maybe views about medication, maybe depression (this is just guesswork, but the GP almost certainly had some hunches) – I'm going to ask them some questions to try to find out more; 'What questions and how do you know their answers will be honest or open or relevant?' – I'll play my hunches and ask questions about those issues. And I don't know – I'm just hoping I might end up knowing a bit more than I know already. And so on, to the point where these questions connect with those posed above: 'How do you know the change in behaviour was significant?'; 'How do you know it was the new strategies that caused the change?' – niggly questions always, but asking 'How do you know?' repeatedly and maintaining that sceptical orientation is an important aspect of any kind of research.

What this example illustrates is how the emphasis of research may vary, with the focus of the research question, on several dimensions, as outlined in Box 3 (overleaf).

On the whole, these dimensions (rigour to relevance, for example) run in parallel with positivist and interpretivist paradigms respectively, but only on the whole. It can be just as misleading to presume that all positivist research is 'reality-based', generalisable and rigorous – concerned to predict and control rather than develop understanding – as to expect that interpretivist research will always involve in-depth study of great relevance and richness – concerned with understanding meanings rather than a desire to influence 'real' events.

**Box 3: Tensions and dimensions – positivist and
interpretivist concerns**

Rigour and relevance

It is easier to achieve rigour if a small number of identified variables are
held constant. This may have the effect, however, of limiting the scope
and richness of exploration. To seek out other potentially relevant
'variables' or aspects of the situation may increase richness and relevance,
but with less control over the procedures. Other forms of rigour (for
example, ensuring that detailed records are kept of encounters and
assumptions throughout) then have to come into play.

Generalisability and differentiation

The main concern may be to ensure that the knowledge gleaned can be
generalised to other situations, that it has some kind of universality in its
implications. On the other hand, the concern may be with understanding
the specifics of the unique case. In the latter case, however, there is likely
to be some presumption of relevance to broader understandings, even if
only by informing future thinking.

Reality and relativism

The research may presume to seek out the truth as far as possible,
enabling accurate predictions about cause and effect to be made.
Alternatively, no one truth may be assumed, but explanations and
meanings may be explored and found to be more or less useful and to
carry more or less weight.

---

4   Who knows? Power and perspectives in research

The third underpinning human concern suggested in Figure 1 was
'to address ethical issues and promote desired values'. Both positivist and
interpretivist traditions operate within such a framework of moral
concern. While hermeneutics and qualitative research engage more
explicitly with values and ethics as an intrinsic part of their subject
matter, the concerns of the researcher are present in traditional scientific
method as well. It would be absurd to suggest that the attempt to remain
neutral in order to test out a hypothesis means that the researcher
therefore has no concern about the potential impact of the findings. The
nature of the value base will, of course, vary and, as Chapter 6 makes clear,
will not always be benign. The recognition that ethical issues and values,
albeit often unrecognised, will affect the conception, progress and analysis
of research is the focus of this final section.

A declaration of bias

In the late 1970s and the 1980s, feminists criticised research in the social sciences in terms of its overarching gender bias. They claimed that most research was the study of men in society and that it was an inherently 'male science of society' (Smith, 1988). This was in effect a two-pronged attack. First, the accusation was that women had largely been ignored – that most research was about the public world of social institutions, work, economic life, crime, and so on. These were areas where women had been traditionally underrepresented. But it was more than that. Not only were women's voices and women's concerns ignored but also there was an assumption that gender was not an issue, whereas for feminists gender relationships and gender divisions were fundamental and defining characteristics that shaped these phenomena in ways that were not being acknowledged.

The second prong of attack is perhaps more complicated. The 'objectivity' of the whole research enterprise was called into question because it was seen to be filtered through a male lens. 'Its whole approach to the study of the social world was coloured by a masculinist bias' (Maynard, 1994). It was a male way of knowing as well as focusing mainly on men. So the remedy was not simply to add in women. It was to redefine what counts as knowledge and to find ways of making that knowledge transparent.

The way to cope with this bias, feminists proposed, was not to try to control or eliminate it, but to make such influences transparent. The researcher thus deliberately acknowledges and reflects on her own history and values. In a series of publications, the feminist philosopher Sandra Harding (1986, 1987, 1991) argues that making the subjective position explicit in this way produces 'strong objectivity' and that there can be no neutral position in the way the scientific method had traditionally proposed.

Part of the concern with breaking down the dichotomy between objectivity and subjectivity is to break down the hierarchical power relationship that has characterised much research. Good feminist research involves gaining the trust of the researched through sharing information and creating a non-exploitative, non-oppressive relationship (see, for example, Johnson, 1998, further discussed in Chapter 4). For many feminist researchers this transformational potential is highly prized (Maynard, 1994). 'Standpoint research', as it has come to be known, involves embracing 'conscious partiality' (Mies, 1983) and has proved to be perhaps the most contentious aspect of feminist research. It also asks who is entitled to be a 'knower' and seems to suggest that only women can be involved in research into women. This orthodoxy did not go unchallenged (Kelly *et al.*, 1994) as black and lesbian women, for example, pointed out that the experiences of women were not homogeneous and that there were significant differences as well as similarities.

Despite such difficulties, feminist research did champion the cause of a particular group in society and 'feel free to substitute explicit interests for implicit ones' (Reinharz, 1985, p. 17). Other oppressed groups in society – disabled people (see, for example, Oliver, 1990; Shakespeare and Watson, 1997; Morris, 1991) and black people (Baxter, 1988; Mama, 1993; Dominelli, 1989) for example – have also seen the importance of taking control of research in order to establish their own research agendas. In doing so they have developed new and more radical interpretations of their circumstances and life experiences.

Research and empowerment

So what does all this tell us about ways of knowing? It tells us that knowledge and the development of knowledge is not value-free. Research is a powerful and power-generating tool that may, wittingly or unwittingly, promote the perspectives and values of the researcher (or the research sponsor) – who is already likely to be in a privileged position. There are, in other words, ways of knowing that will serve to shore up the status quo. Feminists, of course, were not the first to notice this. Marxist research, for example, was similarly involved in making choices designed to champion the cause of oppressed people.

One route to such empowerment has seen research 'subjects' becoming research 'participants' or 'researchers' in their own right. Participatory research has its roots in the radical thinking of Paulo Freire, a Brazilian whose focus was also the emancipation of oppressed groups. Freire (1972, for example) argues that, to be liberated from oppression, people need to acquire a critical awareness of the world in which they live and the structures that surround them. Only then can they act to transform their world. This involves having control over setting the agenda – the problem posing as well as the problem solving (Freire, 1972).

Even if full emancipation from oppression is a remote dream, there are ethical arguments for seeking to develop the ways in which research can empower service-users in health and social care contexts. Narrowing the gap between 'lay' and 'expert' knowledge, supporting service-user research initiatives and challenges, making research-related information more available and accessible, widening and informing debates about health and social care and creating people-sensitive research priorities must contribute in some way to developing fairer and more accountable services.

For researchers and professionals trained in conventional educational methods, the leap from telling people what to do, in their best interests, to welcoming and supporting challenges to professional knowledge can be an uncomfortable one. For health professionals trained within a medical model, who are used to giving advice and supervising treatment, it can be particularly difficult. As Andrea Cornwall explains, the use of participatory methods:

... demands a style of interaction and a change in approach that in itself opens up transformational possibilities. By bringing health professionals into communities, to learn from rather than to teach people, participatory methods open up spaces for dialogue. This experience can be humbling for health workers. Realizing that people are not only knowledgeable but also capable of generating their own solutions has, for many, been a revelation. Working together with local people, as counterparts, challenges deeply held prejudices about the poor.

(Cornwall, 1996, p. 104)

This sharing and shifting of knowledge and power is not without its problems. Democratising decision making is not straightforward. Local people do not speak with one voice and, as feminist standpoint researchers found, the differences between a group of people identified on the basis of one socio-economic category, such as women, can contain many different and conflicting voices. Categories such as 'the oppressed' or 'the poor' can hide immense variations in the experience and needs of different individuals. Resolving conflict and building consensus remains a challenge within participatory research. It is a challenge that has to be met if the interests of stakeholders are to influence the policies and practices that structure their lives.

The climate, which has nurtured participatory research and the breaking down of barriers in terms of who can be knowers, has also nurtured a breaking down of barriers between research methodologies. Standpoint theory opens up the possibility that there are multiple viewing positions and multiple realities, that 'ways of knowing are inherently culture-bound and perspectival' (Lather, 1988, p. 570). Post-modernism has taken the challenge further in terms of the whole notion of 'the truth'. As Bauman puts it:

Postmodernity ... does not seek to substitute one truth for another, one ideal for another. Instead, it splits the truth, the standards and the ideal into already deconstructed and about to be deconstructed. It denies in advance the right of all and any revelation to slip into the place vacated by the deconstructed/discredited rules. It braces itself for a life without truths, standards and ideals.

(Bauman, 1992, p. ix)

This view of the world can be experienced as nihilistic and result in a post-modern paralysis. What is the point of doing research if the project is doomed from the start and there are no realities out there anyway? And how can it be justified?

If all that research can do is produce multiple, competing versions of the world, it is difficult to see why taxpayers' money should be spent on it. Novelists, poets, leader writers and armchair theorists can all produce versions of the world more cheaply.

(Murphy and Dingwall, 1998, pp. 131–2)

And where does this leave the beleaguered professional who is urged to provide evidence for their every move? Perhaps more importantly, the 'realities' of poverty, illness and social exclusion are real enough to the people experiencing them.

This scepticism seems in the 1990s to have led to a situation where it is more widely accepted that there are competing and only partial 'truths'. This opens up the possibility of researching in a pluralistic way, drawing on different methodological traditions. Such 'triangulation' allows evidence gathered in more than one way to be combined to give, the argument goes, a more precise and illuminating picture. Four main arguments for such pluralism are shown in Box 4.

Box 4: Broadening the research picture

- Investigator triangulation: will another researcher find another side to the story?

- Theory triangulation: are there different ways of thinking about what might be going on here?

- Triangulating the data in terms of time, space and person: will the story be different on another day, in another place, with a different person?

- Methodological triangulation: will different methods shed a different light on things?

Such points reflect the same concerns as listed in Box 3 in that they seek to achieve the best of all worlds: both rigour and relevance; both generalisability and differentiation; both reality and relativity. Of course, resource constraints being what they are, such opportunities for triangulation will be strictly within bounds. Also, while they may lead to fresh insights (Kellaher et al., 1990), they may lead to equally fresh confusions (Hammersley and Atkinson, 1983). Indeed, Bloor (1997) argues that we should be very sceptical about any claim to triangulation as the basis of a 'truer' picture. What the arguments for triangulation do not quite take on board, furthermore, is that 'ways of knowing' include more than just research evidence. Practitioners come to know through absorbing and reflecting a wide array of inputs and experiences. Their practice will depend on their theoretical understandings and their experience as well as their grasp of research-based knowledge. It is right and appropriate that such 'knowing' should be open to challenge and the explicit and accountable nature of research puts it in pole position to bring a sceptical and critical gaze to what is offered in the name of health and social care. At the same time, research itself needs to be the object of scrutiny and the different influences to which it is subject need to be borne in mind.

By understanding the strengths and limitations of different approaches across the broad methodological field, practitioners will be able to bring a critical eye to their interpretation of research findings. They can deliberately search out studies that use different methods and stem from different traditions and consider them in relation to each other and in relation to the underpinning concerns that may have motivated the research. Ways of knowing, however, will continue to be influenced by informal as well as formal processes. Recognising this, and being able to value as well as critique their own assumptions, may enable practitioners to engage more fully and positively with the new emphasis on evidence-based practice.

Conclusion

Knowing that the answer to everything is 42, as Deep Thought revealed, is not likely to get anyone very far, although practitioners in health and social care may be forgiven for wishing that sometimes the answers were that simple!

Knowledge is essentially context and purpose specific and evolves through complex and interacting mechanisms, both formal and informal. Political and power dimensions as well as socio-cultural influences will affect how knowing develops. Knowing how to deliver a baby, prevent TB, reduce reoffending or best support single teenage mothers are not just matters of opinion, nor do they just involve developing the theoretical and technical base of knowledge, skill and understanding. Knowing, or coming to know, involves an ongoing transformative struggle to establish itself alongside other vested interests or conflicting moral and political positions. New knowledge is often treated as heresy. Knowing may also involve multiple layers of understanding of which knowing how to implement or act upon knowing may be a crucial element.

There are many ways of knowing. Making choices about how to find out more will depend on what we want to know and why and on our values and assumptions about how best to find out. Awareness of research methodologies can refine and strengthen both formal and informal knowing if it is based on a respectful, broad and self-critical understanding of theories of knowing. Knowledge is power and the privileging of research knowledge as a way of knowing can be tempered by bearing in mind the purposes to which knowledge may be put.

References

Adams, D. (1979) *The Hitch Hiker's Guide to the Galaxy*, London, Pan Books.

Bauman, Z. (1992) *Intimations of Post Modernity*, London, Routledge.

Baxter, C. (1988) *The Black Nurse: An Endangered Species*, Cambridge, Training in Health and Race.

Bloor, M. (1997) 'Techniques of validation in qualitative research: a critical commentary', in Miller, G. and Dingwall, R. (eds) *Context and Method in Qualitative Research*, pp. 37–50, London, Sage.

Bowlby, J. (1988) *A Secure Base*, London, Routledge.

Cooper, N., Stevenson, C. and Hale, G. (1996) *Integrating Perspectives on Health*, Buckingham, Open University Press.

Cornwall, A. (1996) 'Towards participatory practice: participatory rural appraisal (PRA) and the participatory process', in de Koning, K. and Martin, M. (eds) *Participatory Research in Health*, pp. 94–107, London, Zed Books.

Crotty, M. (1998) *The Foundations of Social Research*, London, Sage.

Dilthey, W. (1976) 'The rise of hermeneutics', in Connerton, P. (ed.) *Critical Psychology: Selected Readings*, Harmondsworth, Penguin.

Dominelli, L. (1989) *Anti-Racist Social Work*, London, BASW/Macmillan.

Finlay, L. (1999) 'Applying phenomenology in research: problems, principles and practice', *British Journal of Occupational Therapy*, Vol. 62, No. 7, pp. 299–306.

Freire, P. (1972) *Pedagogy of the Oppressed*, London, Sheed Ward.

Gergen, K. and Gergen, M. (1991) 'Towards reflexive methodologies', in Steier, F. (ed.) *Research and Reflexivity*, London, Sage.

von Glaserfield, E. (1991) 'Knowing without metaphysics: aspects of the radical constructivist position', in Steier, F. (ed.) *Research and Reflexivity*, London, Sage.

Goffman, E. (1968) *Asylums*, Harmondsworth, Pelican Books.

Habermas, J. (1972) *Knowledge and Human Interest*, London, Heinemann.

Hammersley, M. and Atkinson, P. (1983) *Ethnography: Principles in Practice*, London, Tavistock.

Harding, S. (1986) *The Science Question in Feminism*, Milton Keynes, Open University Press.

Harding, S. (1987) *Feminism and Methodology*, Milton Keynes, Open University Press.

Harding, S. (1991) *Whose Science? Whose Knowledge?*, Ithaca, New York, Cornell University Press.

Harré, R. (1986) (ed.) *The Social Construction of Emotions*, Oxford, Basil Blackwell.

Heidegger, M. (1962) *Being and Time*, Oxford, Basil Blackwell.

Hughes, J. (1990) *The Philosophy of Social Research*, London, Longman.

Johnson, K. (1998) *Deinstitutionalising Women: An Ethnographic Study of Institutional Closure*, Cambridge, Cambridge University Press.

Kellaher, L., Peace, S. and Willcocks, D. (1990) 'Triangulating data', in Peace, S. (ed.) *Research Social Gerontology*, London, Sage.

Kelly, L., Barton, S. and Regan, L. (1994) 'Researching women's lives or studying women's oppression? Reflections on what constitutes feminist research', in Maynard, M. and Purvis, J. (eds) *Researching Women's Lives from a Feminist Perspective*, London, Taylor and Francis.

Lather, P. (1988) *Issues of Validity in Openly Ideological Research: Between a Rock and a Soft Place*, London, Interchange.

Mama, A. (1993) 'Violence against black women: gender, race and state responses', in Walmsley, J. *et al.* (eds) *Health, Welfare and Practice: Reflecting on Roles and Relationships*, London, Sage in association with The Open University (K263 reader).

Maynard, M. (1994) 'Methods, practice and epistemology', in Maynard, M. and Purvis, J. (eds) *Researching Women's Lives from a Feminist Perspective*, London, Taylor and Francis.

Menzies, I. (1960) 'A case study in the functioning of social systems as a defence against anxiety: a report on the nursing service of a general hospital', *Human Relations*, pp. 95–121.

Mies, M. (1983) 'Towards a methodology for feminist research', in Bowles, G. and Duelli-Klein, R. (eds) *Theories of Women's Studies*, London, Routledge and Kegan Paul.

Morris, J. (1991) *Pride Against Prejudice*, London, Women's Press.

Murphy, E. and Dingwall, R. (1998) 'Qualitative methods in health services research', in Black, N., Brazier, J., Fitzpatrick, R. and Reeves, B. (eds) *Methods for Health Care Research*, pp. 129–38, London, BMJ Books.

Oliver, M. (1990) *The Politics of Disablement*, London, Macmillan.

Popper, K. R. (1959) *The Logic of Scientific Discovery*, New York, Basic Books.

Popper, K. R. (1963) *Conjectures and Refutations: The Growth of Scientific Discovery*, London, Routledge and Kegan Paul.

Potter, J. (1996) *Representing Reality: Discourse, Rhetoric and Social Construction*, London, Sage.

Reinharz, S. (1985) *Feminist Distruct: A Response to Misogyny and Gynopia in Sociological Work*, unpublished manuscript.

Shakespeare, T. and Watson, N. (1997) 'Defending the social model', *Disability and Society*, Vol. 12, No. 2, pp. 293–300.

Shotter, J. and Gergen, K. (1989) (eds) *Texts of Identity*, London, Sage.

Smith, D. (1988) 'A peculiar eclipsing', in Smith, D. (ed.) *The Everyday World as Problematic: A Feminist Sociology*, Milton Keynes, Open University Press.

Thompson, N. (1995) *Theory and Practice in Health and Social Welfare*, Buckingham, Open University Press.

Usher, R. (1997) 'Introduction', in McKenzie, G., Powell, J. and Usher, R. (eds) *Understanding Social Research: Perspectives on Methodology and Practice*, London, Falmer Press.

Warnke, B. (1987) *Gadamer: Hermeneutics, Tradition and Reason*, Cambridge, Polity Press.

Weber, M. (1962) *Basic Concepts in Sociology*, London, Peter Owen.

Workman, C. (1998) *Adherence Considerations in Primary Care*, paper presented to 12th World Aids Conference, Geneva.

Chapter 2
Making sense of surveys

Roger Gomm

Introduction

Most people contribute to a survey at some time during their life: on a street corner; responding to a junk mail-shot; or giving permission for details in their social work records to be extracted anonymously for research purposes. Whatever the purpose of the survey (Box 1), the quality of the data depends on how well the survey was designed and executed and how well it serves the purpose for which it was designed.

> **Box 1: Some uses of surveys in research relevant to health and social care**
>
> - Gauging levels of satisfaction with services among service-users
> - Ascertaining public support for different policy options – see Chapter 11
> - Evaluating the effect of an intervention – for example, collecting data about health-related attitudes in an area which has been subjected to a health education campaign, and in an area which has not (Tudor-Smith *et al.*, 1998)
> - Monitoring agency performance or policy implementation
> - Collecting data within an experimental strategy – see Chapter 3
> - Needs assessment through a community survey
> - Ethnic and gender monitoring
> - Charting the distribution of some phenomenon, geographically and within a population – for example, the regional distribution of drug misuse, the social class distribution of domestic violence, the ethnic distribution of health-related behaviours.

The key question in this chapter is 'What makes a survey believable?' But it will also illustrate much about what makes any kind of quantitative research believable by using the topic of surveys to illustrate the four main criteria used to judge technical quality.

- **Validity** – do the results accurately reflect what it is claimed they reflect?

- **Reliability** – were the results free from the kinds of distortions that arise from using inconsistent methods?

- **Representativeness** and **generalisability** – are the findings true only of what was studied, or would they be true more widely?

- **Fitness for purpose** – were the methods used fit for the purpose of the research?

1 Comparing two surveys

The discussion will be illustrated with a case study of two consumer satisfaction surveys of the NHS based on work by Cohen *et al.* (1996). The surveys were done at much the same time and place but they have different results. Why should this be so? What does it tell us about the criteria listed above? And what lessons does this have for practitioners in health and social care trying to make sense of survey research findings?

Consumer satisfaction with the NHS in Scotland

Table 1 (overleaf) compares the results of two patient satisfaction surveys in Scotland. The NHS Users' Survey is an all-Scotland survey conducted once in 1992/3 and once in 1993/4 (National Health Service in Scotland, 1993, 1994; Capewell, 1994). The results are pooled in the table. The other is a survey in the Lothian Region in 1993 (Cohen *et al.*, 1994).

The table shows *dis*-satisfaction rates. Thus the first figure in the table shows that, in the Lothian Survey, 96.6% (100 minus 3.4%) had no complaints to make about 'respect for patients' privacy'. Aspects 8, 9 and 10 pose a puzzle. Do these large differences arise because the health services in Lothian are different from those in Scotland as a whole, or because the people in Lothian expect more of the NHS than do people in Scotland generally? Or does something about the way in which the two surveys were conducted account for the differences? These questions will be explored throughout the rest of this chapter.

Table 1   **Patient dissatisfaction rates in two population surveys: patients with recent hospital experience (figures are age-weighted percentages of respondents)**

Aspect of patient care	Lothian Health Survey (1993)	NHS Users' Survey (1992–4)
1 Respect for patients' privacy	3.4%	2.7%
2 Respect for patients' dignity	3.2%	3.0%
3 Sensitivity to patients' feelings	6.3%	5.2%
4 Treated as an individual or a whole person	9.0%	5.7%
5 Treated like a child and patronised	10.6%	–
6 Clear explanation of care or enough information	8.7 %	7.1%
7 Understanding of what doctor is saying	6.4%	2.4%
8 Encouraged to ask questions*	23.9%	5.6%
9 Given time to ask questions or be involved*	12.5%	3.9%
10 Listened to by doctors or staff*	12.5%	3.2%
Total sample size†	2058	2685

* Statistical tests showed that the differences between the Lothian Survey and the NHS Users' Survey were highly statistically significant at p<0.01, which means that less than once in 100 times would differences of this size be expected to occur by chance (Coolican, 1994, pp. 234–52).

† The adult population living in the community was surveyed in both surveys, but the data here are just for respondents with recent in-patient or out-patient hospital experience.

(Source: based on Cohen *et al.*, 1996, p. 842)

Statistically significant differences

The differences between the two surveys on aspects 8, 9 and 10 are *statistically significant*. Testing for statistical significance means comparing what was actually found with what might have happened by chance. If the actual results were very unlikely to have occurred by chance, the results are said to be statistically significant. In this case, the test resulted in a figure of p<0.01. The p stands for probability. It is less than 0.01. This means that this result would be expected to have happened by chance less than once in 100 times. But less than once in 100 times of what?

The logic of statistical testing rests on the idea of repeated random sampling. Consider topic 8 in Table 1. This gives a figure of 23.9% for the Lothian Survey and 5.6% for the NHS Users' Survey. The question a statistician asks is 'What is the chance of samples with these values being drawn from the *same* population?' Since there are no better data on which to base an estimate, this hypothetical 'same' population is assumed to have a dissatisfaction rate of the two samples combined: about 14%. Intuitively, you know that if you continued drawing random samples of around 2000 from such a population then a large percentage of them would show dissatisfaction rates fairly close to the 14% norm, say between 12.5 and 15.5%. Some samples would crop up with rates below 12.5 and above 15.5% but these would be rare. The statistical test puts a number to this rarity at less than 1% for any such samples (less than 0.01). Since the actual values in Table 1 would only very rarely crop up by chance, it is reasonable to assume that they are not drawn from a single population with a dissatisfaction rate of 14%, but from two different populations with different dissatisfaction rates. That is what a statistically significant difference means.

The same principle also allows for the calculation of *sampling errors*, or *confidence intervals*. This is what archaeologists express when they say '4000 BC plus or minus 550 years'. Although not shown in Table 1, there would be confidence intervals for all these figures, saying in effect that 'the best estimate is the figure given, but the true figure might be plus or minus this'. The most usual errors/intervals quoted are the 95% or the 99% errors/intervals, meaning that 95% or 99% of all random samples would be expected to fall between these two points.

In Table 1 only three aspects give statistically significant differences. For the others, the two surveys give different figures but of a size that might often have arisen by chance in drawing random samples from the same population. There is no point in thinking up more elaborate explanations for these differences, when chance alone is enough to explain them.

2 Explaining the differences

So far, then, some differences between the two surveys have been eliminated as uninteresting. But there are still three sets of results showing statistically significant differences. They need explaining.

Real differences or research artefacts?

Research methods shape research results so it is useful to know precisely how different research techniques work to produce the results they do. This also puts a premium on researchers reporting the methods used in enough detail to allow others to replicate the research or, more usually, to think through the production process, to audit it, to see how the results were produced.

Are the differences highlighted in Table 1 *real* differences or are they *artefacts* of the methods used? The terms 'real' and 'artefact' are somewhat slippery, so it is better to rephrase the question to ask 'Where in the research process are these differences coming from?' Some options are suggested in Box 2 (overleaf). Conventionally, options 1, 2 and 3 would be regarded as real differences, and 4 and 5 as artefacts: 4 as a sampling artefact and 5 as an instrumental or a measurement artefact.

> **Box 2: Some possible sources of the statistically significant differences between the NHS Users' Survey and the Lothian Survey**
>
> *Option 1.* There are differences in the performance of health services in Lothian by comparison with Scotland as a whole. These are reflected in the differences between surveys.
>
> OR
>
> *Option 2.* No differences of the kind above but the population structure of Lothian is uncharacteristic of the population of Scotland in a way that influences the rate of dissatisfaction.
>
> OR
>
> *Option 3.* No differences of the kinds above but the people in Lothian have higher expectations of the health service than the people in Scotland as a whole. This is what is shown in the differences between the surveys.
>
> OR
>
> *Option 4.* No differences of the kinds above, but the Lothian sample over-represented, or the all-Scotland sample under-represented, dissatisfied patients in each location. This is what shows up as the difference between the two surveys. This would be a sampling artefact and an issue of representativeness.
>
> OR
>
> *Option 5.* No differences of any of the kinds above, but the two surveys asked questions in different ways, yielding different answers and this accounts for the difference. This would be an instrumental artefact.

One version of Option 2 can be deleted immediately. Lothian does have a younger population than Scotland as a whole. Younger people are more likely to express dissatisfaction with the NHS. But the figures in Table 1 are *age-weighted*. They have been recalculated as if the two populations had an identical age structure (Cohen *et al.*, 1996, p. 842). Any effect of age differences between the two populations has been controlled for, so there is no real difference here.

Sampling and representativeness

In a *sample survey* a sample is selected to stand for or *represent* the *population of interest*. In Table 1 this population is all adults living in the community in the respective areas who had recent hospital experience. Both the Scottish NHS surveys used *probability* to select a sample. This means that, as far as possible, everyone in the population had an equal chance of being selected and that the selection was made by some random principle such as using a table of random numbers. Nearly all methodology textbooks contain detailed information about techniques of sample selection (for example, Bowling, 1997; Alston and Bowles, 1998; Arber, 1993).

The representativeness of a probability sample is vulnerable in three main ways.

1 Not everyone in the population of interest will have an equal chance of being selected. For Lothian the starting point, or *sampling frame*, was a listing of all people registered with a GP, excluding about 4% of the population.

2 Not all those selected will be surveyed. Some will refuse, not be contactable, or be too ill to participate. In the all-Scotland survey this *non-response* was 20%; in Lothian it was 22%. Non-responses above 25% should begin to raise suspicions about the representativeness of a sample.

3 There is non-response at the level of individual questions in a questionnaire: some people do not answer all the questions. In opinion surveys that use open-ended questions (rather than forced-choice questions), there is the obverse problem. Some people give more answers to a question than do others, biasing the results towards the views of the more loquacious.

It is the make-up, not the size, of the non-respondent group that is important (Arber, 1993, pp. 83–86). Only if the people excluded were very different from those included, in ways relevant to the research, would this seriously undermine the sample's representativeness. In the Lothian Survey there were significantly lower response rates from the poorest wards. Hence the survey was biased towards expressing the opinions of better-off people. In both surveys younger people were more likely to be non-respondents than older ones (Cohen *et al.*, 1996, p. 842). Survey researchers usually cross-check the representativeness of the group who actually do respond against known characteristics of the population from which they are drawn. These might be characteristics such as the population's age profile or its sex ratio. If samples are representative of their populations for known factors, it is reasonable to assume they will be representative for some as yet unknown ones too.

Samples, however, are never simply representative. They will be representative in some respects and not in others. At over 2000, the sample size for the all-Scotland results in Table 1 would be big enough to include around 50 black and Asian people, who make up less than 2% of the adult population of Scotland. This would be too small a sample to give an accurate representation of the sex ratio within the minority ethic population, let alone to represent differences *among* black and Asian people in terms of their experience of the NHS. *Stratification by ethnicity* would be necessary to recruit an adequate minority sample for this. A stratified sample (sometimes termed a weighted sample) over-represents some groups in the sample by comparison with the percentage of the population they constitute. This is in order to recruit a sufficient number for their characteristics or opinions to be surveyed.

The possibility of a sampling artefact

Table 1 deals only with people who had recent experience of hospitals. There are over 2000 of these for each survey. They are treated as just three kinds of people: those who agreed with a statement; those who disagreed; or those who did not know/would not say. For representing this low level of diversity the sample sizes are huge. The smaller the degree of diversity a survey attempts to represent, the less effect non-response will have in skewing the results away from representativeness.

Cohen and his colleagues checked the samples against what was known about the populations from which they were drawn and concluded that the results of both surveys are probably biased by non-response. The data particularly under-represent the views of younger people, who are known to be more likely to express dissatisfaction (Bosanquet and Zarzecka, 1995, p. 89). But because the bias is of the same magnitude and in the *same* direction in *both* surveys, this cannot explain the *differences* in the results (Cohen *et al.*, 1996, p. 843).

Representativeness and generalisability

Sampling artefacts have consequences for the confidence with which generalisations can be made from samples to the populations from which they were drawn.

What is generalised from a sample to a population is a *frequency distribution*. The generalisation might be:

> Since approximately 9 out of 10 people *in the sample* were satisfied with the NHS, it will also be true that approximately 9 out of 10 people in the adult population of Scotland, living in the community, with recent hospital experience, will be satisfied.

Usually such generalisations are given with confidence intervals: an estimate plus or minus something. Most of the figures in Table 1 can be regarded as estimates plus or minus no more than 2%. Big samples give precise estimates. But this precision applies only to the extent that the samples were fully representative. The incompleteness of the sampling frame and the non-response will make the estimates less accurate than this.

Here neither survey is *fully* representative at the chosen level of representativeness for the population from which it is drawn. Few samples ever are. Generalisations from both have to be issued with a warning saying that, compared with opinion in the unsurveyed population, both samples probably exaggerate the degree of satisfaction with the NHS, although not by a huge degree.

For explaining the differences between the surveys, a sampling artefact explanation is probably ruled out, although it remains a possibility that in over-representing the views of better-off people, the Lothian Survey over-represented dissatisfied patients, since better-off people usually express more dissatisfaction with the NHS (Bosanquet and Zarzecka, 1995, p. 89). However, if artefacts are important here, they are probably the kind resulting from the instruments used: from the way questions were asked, for example.

Measurement or instrumental artefacts

The ideal way to investigate how an instrument shapes the data collected is to use a second instrument to collect data from the same people and compare the two results. This is routine practice with measurement devices used in experimental research. Thermometers are calibrated against other thermometers; scales measuring depression are validated against other scales measuring depression or by panels of clinicians (Jenkinson, 1994). In looking for explanations for the differences between the surveys, it would have been ideal to have administered the Lothian questionnaire to the respondents of the NHS Users' Survey and vice versa. However, this would have been impractical and very expensive, and the results would have been confounded by the passage of time. What Cohen and his colleagues could and did do was to look at the responses given by people in Lothian to the NHS Users' Survey, which, of course, covered Lothian as well as the rest of Scotland. This allowed them to ask whether people from Lothian were also more dissatisfied in the answers they had given to the questions in the all-Scotland NHS Users' Survey.

The results are shown in Table 2 (overleaf). This repeats what was shown in Table 1: for three topics there are statistically significant differences between all the people surveyed in the Lothian Survey and all the people surveyed in the NHS Users' Survey. But the extra column shows that when people from Lothian had answered questions on the NHS Users' Survey, there was no significant difference between their answers and those of people elsewhere in Scotland. This was true not only for the three issues but also for all the issues shown in Table 1 (Cohen *et al.*, 1996, p. 842). This pin-points the reason for the differences being something about the way the questions were either administered or framed.

Table 2   **Patient dissatisfaction rates in two population surveys: showing that the responses of people in Lothian to the NHS Users' Survey were similar to those of other people in Scotland in the same survey but different from responses in the Lothian Survey**

Aspect of patient care	Lothian Health Survey (1993)	NHS Users' Survey (1992–4)	Lothian sub-sample of NHS Users' Survey †
Encouraged to ask questions*	23.9%	5.6%	4.2%
Given time to ask questions or be involved*	12.5%	3.9%	3.1%
Listened to by doctors or staff*	12.5%	3.2%	2.3%
Total sample size	2058	2685	310

* Statistical tests showed that the differences between the Lothian Survey and the NHS Users' Survey were highly statistically significant at $p<0.01$, which means that less than once in 100 times would differences of this size be expected to occur by chance (Coolican, 1994, pp. 234–52).

† There were no statistically significant differences between the Lothian sub-sample of the NHS Users' Survey and the all-Scotland results from the NHS Users' Survey.

(Source: based on Cohen *et al.*, 1996, p. 842)

The NHS Users' Survey was administered face-to-face in a 30-minute interview. The Lothian Survey was a self-completed postal questionnaire. It was the Lothian Survey that elicited the higher level of dissatisfaction. Perhaps the anonymity of a postal questionnaire empowered respondents to be more critical. Perhaps the face-to-face situation of the NHS Users' Survey inhibited the articulation of criticism. Open-ended questions, which leave it up to respondents to raise dissatisfactions, yield much lower rates of dissatisfaction than do forced-choice questions offering opportunities to express dissatisfaction (Locker and Dunt, 1978). But both these surveys used forced-choice questionnaires.

There were also important differences in the questions and the questioning strategy (Table 3).

Cohen *et al.* (1996, p. 843) comment:

Whereas only 5.6% of respondents in the Scottish users' survey agreed with the statement "I was not encouraged to ask questions", 23.9% of the Lothian respondents disagreed with the statement "You were encouraged to ask questions about your treatment." Thus substantially different conclusions can be obtained if patients are presented with a negative statement about care and asked to agree that something "bad" happened, as opposed to presenting them with a positive statement and asking them to disagree that something "good" happened.

Table 3 **Differences in questioning strategy and wording between the Lothian and the NHS Users' Surveys**

Lothian Survey	NHS Users' Survey
The questionnaire asks:	The *interviewer* asks:
'Thinking generally about your experience in hospital in the last year, please tell us if you agree or disagree with the statements below':	'Thinking about the information you were given at the hospital, did any of these things happen at your visit?'
(for example)	The interviewer displays a card with several negative statements on it:
'You were encouraged to ask questions about your treatment.'	(for example)
And the questionnaire asks:	'I was not given enough information.'
	'I was not encouraged to ask questions.'
'The National Health Service in Scotland published a booklet called *Framework for Action.* They listed some of the things that upset patients. In your experience of hospitals in Lothian are any of these things a cause of concern?'	'I was not encouraged to get involved in decisions about my treatment.'
	'There was not enough time for me to be involved.'
(for example)	Respondents were then asked to indicate the seriousness of any problem they identify in agreeing with a statement, by rating it on a five-point scale.
'Doctors who have no time to listen.'	
'Doctors who ignore what you say.'	

Methodology texts often warn against 'leading questions' in questionnaires. But all questions are 'leading'; some more than others, but they all lead towards an answer. As this example shows, two different wordings might lead in different directions. Cohen *et al.* conclude that the effect may be specific to particular kinds of topic, but research artefacts of this instrumental kind do seem to account best for the differences in results between the two surveys.

3 Reliability in survey research

Weighing the same package twice within a short period of time and getting different results is the mark of an *unreliable* weighing machine. Punctilious survey researchers trial questions with different wordings with the *same* respondents before they decide on a final version. In survey research a reliable approach means gathering data in the same way from every respondent.

Consistency is prioritised. Everyone is confronted with the same questionnaire. Interviewers attempt to behave in the same way towards each respondent. If there are several interviewers, they are trained to

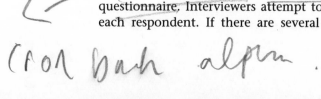
Cron bach alpha.

behave similarly. In large survey research organisations the responses are analysed interviewer by interviewer as a way of estimating whether any difference between interviewers is contaminating the results, just as in examination systems the marks of different examiners are analysed to see whether any are marking higher or lower than the others. All this should ensure that the differences and similarities shown in the results are differences and similarities between respondents and not between interviewers, interviews, different ways of asking questions, and so on (Alreck and Settle, 1995).

Some surveys do not collect information in quite this way. For example, epidemiological surveys are designed to chart the distribution of illnesses or social problems in a population. Here it is usual for medical experts to make and record diagnoses, or social workers to conduct and record assessments. But again the procedures and the criteria for the judgements should be standardised, and the protocols made available to readers of the research (Barker and Rose, 1993, pp. 32–37).

Neither of the Scottish surveys seems to have been marked by any serious unreliability but the example does show that small differences in question wording can give large differences in response. Questioning respondents differently in the *same* survey is likely to have serious consequences.

Modern survey procedures have developed since the 1940s to overcome problems that include judgemental inconsistency by diagnosticians and 'interviewer effects'. The problem with the more traditional, less structured, less standardised, more open-ended approaches was that the responses of interviewees were repeatedly found to reflect more about the interviewers than about the interviewees. An often-quoted example is the huge Kinsey reports on human sexuality (Kinsey *et al.*, 1948, 1953; O'Connell-Davidson and Layder, 1994, pp. 83–113). Kinsey believed that having sex with animals was widespread but that sex between adults and children was very rare. Kinsey himself spent much more time with respondents who reported bestiality than with those who reported child sex abuse. Inevitably, the findings in the Kinsey reports reflect Kinsey's own opinions on this. In political opinion polling, the tendency for respondents to mirror the political opinions of their interviewers has been shown to be very strong if there are no adequate safeguards against this (Finkel *et al.*, 1991). Political opinion polling is very similar to the kinds of health and social care research that elicits the preferences of clients for particular kinds of service, or their satisfactions or dissatisfactions.

The weight of research into research in this field suggests that the less the interviewee can guess about the identity and beliefs of the interviewer, the more accurate the answers will be (Bradburn, 1983). However, what respondents say can only be verified if the questions are about matters of fact: for example, whether they are employed or not, or how many pints of beer they drink per week (Cook and Allen, 1983; Crawford, 1987). But many surveys seek to elicit opinions, feelings or interpretations. Here there are no means of verification.

There have also been problems in international epidemiological research where diagnosticians in different countries work with different definitions of 'the same' illness. National survey research into numbers of children 'at risk' inspires little confidence since different social work teams and areas seem to define 'at risk' differently (Packman *et al.*, 1986; Campbell, 1991).

The way a question is posed will always shape the response. It is unavoidable. Two features of survey research minimise the seriousness of this.

1 If every respondent receives the same questions, any differences between respondents will be due to their different responses to this similarity of treatment. By contrast, in unstructured interviewing each respondent is likely to be treated in a different way. It will be unclear whether any response differences are due to differences between respondents or differences in the way they were interviewed.

2 Standardised questions, often written protocols for interviewers, and sometimes interviewers' field notes or logs, make it much easier for researchers, and people reading the research, to see how response patterns can be attributed to the questioning – as in the case study for this chapter.

Standardised questioning does not eliminate an *interviewer effect*. For example, Nathanson (1978) showed that men reported higher levels of morbidity when they were interviewed by women than when interviewed by men. But this is made knowable by the standardised nature of the questioning and the high level of accountability of survey research. Similarly, unless the results of unstructured research are recorded, transcribed and made available to readers, it is virtually impossible to ascertain how the performance of the interviewer shaped the respondent's answers.

Reliability and comparative judgements

Rudat (1994) found that over 87% of the general population were happy with the outcome of their GP consultation, but only 80% of African-Caribbean, Indian and Pakistani people and only 75% of Bangladeshi people were satisfied. This finding only has credibility and practical implications because all the respondents were asked the same questions in the same way and because samples of each were drawn from their respective populations similarly. This illustrates the importance of using reliable methods wherever comparisons are being made. Comparisons may be between sub-groups of the population, as above, or between points in time. Table 4 (overleaf) shows the results of another consumer survey, repeated in 1983, 1989 and 1993 (Bosanquet and Zarzecka, 1995). It reveals a pattern of declining satisfaction for all respondents, but increasing satisfaction for those who actually experienced in-patient care. This would probably be invisible if *different* surveys had been used in each survey year, or in small-scale, open-ended research.

Table 4   Satisfaction and dissatisfaction with in-patient care: British Social Attitudes Survey – England, Scotland and Wales*

	Percentage satisfied			Percentage dissatisfied			Mean level of satisfaction†		
	1983	1989	1993	1983	1989	1993	1983	1989	1993
All*	73.7	65.4	63.8	6.6	15.4	14.0	3.9	3.5	3.6
Scotland*	80.8	69.5	66.4	7.4	7.2	18.7	3.9	3.6	3.6
Without in-patient experience (all)	NA	64.5	56.2	NA	13.2	14.1	NA	3.4	3.4
With in-patient experience (all)	NA	71.1	72.1	NA	18.3	13.9	NA	3.7	3.8

* Includes both people who had and people who had not experienced in-patient care. The last row of the table shows that those who actually experienced in-patient care show a higher rate of satisfaction which increases over time.

† Respondents were asked to rate their satisfaction on a five-point scale (5 = very satisfied). The mean level of satisfaction is the average score on this scale: satisfied = 4 and 5; dissatisfied = 1 and 2.

(Source: Bosanquet and Zarzecka, 1995, p. 92)

Again, when Lewis and Wilkinson (1993) were investigating the influence of economic recession on mental health, it was important for them to use a survey instrument which had frequently been used in the past. Making comparisons through reliable means is not only important in surveys. It is also important in collecting data for experimental approaches (see Chapter 3).

It would not make much sense to say that the Scottish Users' Survey *under-recorded* patient dissatisfaction, or that the Lothian survey *exaggerated* it, or that the British Social Attitudes Survey (Table 4) exaggerated it even more. The more sensible statement is that the three surveys give *different* measures of satisfaction. For any of them the differences recorded by the same survey between two points in time, or between two sub-groups, would indicate something real. There are difficulties in comparing the results of one survey with another. But these are not so acute as those that arise in comparing the results of two different studies using unstructured interviews.

Similar remarks apply in epidemiological research. Defining any disease or social problem entails making a threshold or 'caseness' decision, answering the question 'What degree of severity distinguishes cases from non-cases?' Thus the National Foundation for Mental Health (1995) puts the prevalence of mental illness at one in four of the population. The OPCS Survey of Psychiatric Morbidity puts it at one in seven (Meltzer *et al.*, 1995). The NFMH research is not particularly rigorous, but in principle there is no reason why two equally well-conducted epidemiological surveys should not result in two different, but equally valid, figures simply because they make different threshold decisions. The same is true in measuring 'abuse', 'racism', 'homelessness', 'at-risk', and so on. When surveys are used as a means of estimating the 'need' for services, different threshold decisions about caseness will feed through to the results of a survey as different estimates of 'need'.

4   Fittingness and validity in survey research

Validity refers to whether research results accurately reflect what it is claimed they reflect. Much hinges then on the researcher's declared intention. All research sets the terms of its own validity (Couvalis, 1997). Claims about validity are really always prefaced by an implied clause which runs: '*If* we define x as such and such *then* ...'. For example: 'If we regard satisfaction with the NHS as what is measured by this questionnaire then ...'

Throughout this book there are examples of trade-offs in research, where choosing a research method that is strong in one respect is choosing a method that is weak in another. Surveys are well suited to produce data that can be quantified so that comparisons can be made between groups within the sample that are *valid* in terms of the way the researcher defines concepts and makes measurements (see also Chapter 3). And they are the best method for charting trends in time through asking the same questions on several different occasions. In so far as the sample was representative, surveys are a good basis for making *valid generalisations* about the distribution of the same phenomena, similarly defined, in the population from which the sample was drawn. However, surveys are rather weak devices for finding out about people's experiences. It is doubtful whether any survey questionnaire could produce valid results if it were prefaced: *If satisfaction means the actual experience of being satisfied as it is lived by each individual then* ... But equally, the kinds of methods used to investigate lived experience are poor in forming the basis for valid comparisons or valid generalisations (see Chapter 4).

Surveys for different uses (Box 1) need to define their terms and make their measurements differently. This will influence what counts as valid. For example, the OPCS survey of psychiatric morbidity concludes that one in seven of the adult population is mentally ill *at any one time* in terms of definitions of mental illness close to those which doctors in practice might use to diagnose a case (Meltzer *et al.*, 1995); although it was designed to find cases irrespective of whether they were known to the services. One purpose was to provide data to judge whether mental health services were adequate to meet needs defined in terms of current medical definitions of mental ill health. A Policy Studies Institute (PSI) survey of the mental health of minority ethnic groups used an approach very similar to the OPCS survey. This was to judge whether minority ethnic groups had higher or lower levels of mental health need, in order to provide a baseline for judging whether mental health services were adequately meeting *these needs, defined thus* (Nazroo, 1997). By contrast with OPCS and PSI, the NFMH preferred its headline figure of one in four of the population experiencing mental illness *during their lifetime*. The purpose was to show that mental illness is normal and widespread and that mental health services need a massive injection of funds. It is not that the OPCS was right and the NFMH was wrong, or vice versa. They were making different kinds of claims for different kinds of purposes. The differences between them are not 'matters of fact' but ethico-political differences in opinion about who-deserves-what, and strategic differences in terms of decisions about what practical actions should be taken.

What, then, might be the use of consumer satisfaction surveys? There is great interest in using sample surveys of this kind to generate performance indicator data to judge the performance of public sector agencies against each other (McIver and Meredith, 1998; Cleary, 1999). For example, several regular surveys on drug and alcohol use are used to monitor the UK Tackling Drugs Together strategy, and the performance of the various agencies implementing it (Cabinet Office, 1999). In 1999 the Department of Health in England instituted annual satisfaction surveys for NHS performance indicator purposes (DoH, 1997). One reason for this is to provide a cross-check on those performance indicators used in the NHS that are based on data supplied by NHS agencies. The quality of these data has been very unsatisfactory to date (Health Service Journal, 1999).

For consumer satisfaction measures to be used in this way they would need to be not so much valid measures of satisfaction as valid measures of performance. An important criterion for a *valid* performance indicator is that it measures performance. When performance changes for better or worse this should be indicated by corresponding changes in the measure. A criterion for a *useful* performance indicator is that it should indicate what managers and practitioners need to do in order to increase their performance indicator score. In health and social care, measures of satisfaction often fail dismally on both counts when treated as performance indicators (Box 3).

As Box 3 suggests, there is no robust relationship between the quality of services provided and how clients rate them. Some difficulties result from the way in which a survey detaches the rating from the experience which allegedly gave rise to it. The problems are less acute with in-house evaluations when it is known what exactly happened to the client, or where client satisfaction is among the outcome measures of an experiment (Chapter 3).

None of the above counts against the value of in-depth investigations of what people want from public services. But satisfaction measures are always of doubtful validity as comparative measures of performance quality because of their grounding in expectations and their sensitivity to factors apart from the treatment received. Recognising this, some consumer surveys do not ask clients for evaluations of service, but instead ask them to answer factual questions: such as whether they have had an operation cancelled or whether they were informed of the results of tests.

Box 3: Why consumer satisfaction is a poor indicator of comparative agency performance

- Almost irrespective of what happens to them, about two-thirds of people will register 'satisfaction' with health or social services. Thus only about one-third of the measuring scale is available for comparing between groups, between services or between points in time (Hall and Dornan, 1988; Wensing *et al.*, 1994). The Lothian questionnaire may be preferable here, since it leaves more 'room for improvement' (Table 1).

- Satisfaction is based on expectations. High satisfaction may indicate high quality services or low expectations developed through experience of poor quality services. Improving services may raise expectations and lower satisfaction levels (Williams, 1994).

- Recall of events and opinions of the 'satisfaction' kind vary greatly according to the mood of the respondent at the time of questioning (Bradburn, 1983).

- There is no necessary relationship between providing what people say they want and their satisfaction with what they receive (for example, Hamm *et al.*, 1996).

- The longer the period that elapses between the experience of services and ratings of satisfaction, the lower the satisfaction expressed. If the time at which the measure is taken is crucial, this adds an important potential for unreliability to measurement (Stimson and Webb, 1975; Savage and Armstrong, 1990).

- Satisfaction measures derived from sample surveys do not relate satisfaction scores to the 'performances' that allegedly gave rise to them. Hence it is difficult for practitioners to know how to respond to them.

- Different social groups show different norms of satisfaction, so the same quality of service will produce different satisfaction ratings according to the make-up of an agency's clientele – as indicated in the earlier discussion (Hall and Dornan, 1990; Bosanquet and Zarzecka, 1995). A ranking of agencies in terms of satisfaction scores is unlikely to be the same as a ranking of agencies in terms of performance judged on other quality criteria.

- Satisfaction with public services is strongly influenced by the mass media, the general 'feel-good' factor, political events such as nurses' strikes, and atrocity stories told by friends and relatives. To a great extent it is outside the control of agencies and practitioners (Carr-Hill, 1992).

This is the approach adopted by the National Survey of Hospital Patients, based on questionnaires previously used in the USA (Bruster *et al.*, 1994).

The way questions are asked will still frame the responses, but the responses to this kind of survey do pin-point areas where service performance is deficient and make it obvious what remedial action is needed.

Thus it appears that satisfaction surveys may be fit for the purpose of making some broad-brush contrasts between the opinions of different social groups, or the same populations at different points in time. But it is a long way from the opinions to the circumstances which gave rise to them. So satisfaction scores are probably not a valid or useful measure of performance.

Conclusion

In a sense all research findings are research artefacts. They are created by research. The important issue is what they were created for and whether they are fit for that purpose.

In order to appraise research it is necessary to do some 'reverse engineering': that is, to dismantle it and see how it was put together. This means translating its claims into operational terms, whether it is survey research or research of any other kind.

Thus the simple statement:

... only 3.4% of adults in Lothian were dissatisfied with the respect shown for patients' privacy in the NHS

needs to be expanded to read:

... in 1993, of a sample of 2058 adults [age-weighted thus ...] who had recent hospital experience ['recent' defined thus ...], drawn from Lothian, using these methods of sampling [...], with a non-response of this size and composition [...], only 3.4% agreed with [this statement] on a self-administered postal questionnaire which we regard as an instrument for measuring satisfaction. It can further be claimed that something near to 3.4% [plus or minus these confidence intervals ...] of the adult population of Lothian, who in 1993 had recent experience of hospital treatment [as already defined], would have responded in the same way to the same question had they been asked it in the same way.

The second sentence of the expanded version is a generalisation. It is a conjecture, as generalisations always are, but a well-informed conjecture, and made accountable in the longer version. The cogency of the generalisation rests on whether the components of the argument fit together logically, and whether the research procedures indicated were adequately carried out. In competent survey research the procedures used are specified in detail (somewhere), so they can be audited by other people. In principle the validity of the generalisation can be checked by repeating the research in as near as possible the same way, although in practice this rarely happens with surveys. Change any one of the major components in the long version and it will make some difference to what would count as a valid generalisation *following from* the research.

The key question for this chapter was 'What makes a survey believable?' The answer is that there are no good grounds for believing or disbelieving survey results unless the researchers provide a detailed account along the lines of the longer version above. Thereafter what makes a survey believable is how well it survives the reader's detailed scrutiny. The same applies to any research findings.

References

Alreck, P. and Settle, R. (1995) *The Survey Research Handbook* (2nd edn), Burr Ridge, Ill., Irwin.

Alston, M. and Bowles, W. (1998) *Research for Social Workers: An Introduction to Methods*, London, Allen and Unwin.

Arber, S. (1993) 'Designing samples', in Gilbert, N. (ed.) *Researching Social Life*, pp. 68–92, London, Sage.

Barker, D. and Rose, G. (1993) *Epidemiology in Medical Practice*, Edinburgh, Churchill Livingstone.

Bosanquet, N. and Zarzecka, A. (1995) 'Attitudes to health services 1983 to 1993', in Harrison, A. and Bruscini, S. (eds) *Health Care UK 1994/95: An Annual Review of Health Care Policy*, pp. 88–94, London, King's Fund Policy Institute.

Bowling, A. (1997) *Research Methods in Health: Investigating Health and Health Services*, Buckingham, Open University Press.

Bradburn, N. (1983) 'Response effects', in Rossi, J., Wright, D. and Anderson, A. (eds) *Handbook of Social Survey Research*, pp. 289–328, New York, Academic Press.

Bruster, S., Jarman, B., Bosanquet, N., Weston, D., Erens, R. and Delbanco, T. (1994) 'National survey of hospital patients', *British Medical Journal*, Vol. 309, pp. 1542–49.

Cabinet Office (1999) *Targets/KPI and Reporting Mechanisms*, London, The UK Anti-Drugs Co-ordination Unit of the Cabinet Office.

Campbell, M. (1991) 'Children at risk: how different are children on child abuse registers?', *British Journal of Social Work*, Vol. 21, pp. 259–75.

Capewell, S. (1994) 'What users think: a survey of NHS users in Scotland in 1992', *Health Bulletin*, Vol. 52, pp. 26–34.

Carr-Hill, R. (1992) 'The measurement of public satisfaction', *Journal of Public Health Medicine*, Vol. 14, No. 3, pp. 236–49.

Cleary, P. (1999) 'The increasing importance of patient surveys', *British Medical Journal*, Vol. 319, pp. 720–1.

Cohen, G., Forbes, J. and Garraway, M. (1994) *Lothian Health Survey – Summary of Initial Findings*, Edinburgh, Edinburgh University Department of Public Health Sciences.

Cohen, G., Forbes, J. and Garraway, M. (1996) 'Can different patient satisfaction surveys yield consistent results? Comparison of three surveys', *British Medical Journal*, Vol. 313, No. 7061, pp. 841–4.

Cook, D. and Allen, C. (1983) 'Self-reported alcohol consumption and dissimulation in a Scottish urban sample', *Journal of Studies on Alcohol*, Vol. 44, pp. 617–29.

Coolican, H. (1994) *Research Methods and Statistics in Psychology* (2nd edn), London, Hodder and Stoughton.

Couvalis, G. (1997) *The Philosophy of Science: Science and Objectivity*, London, Sage.

Crawford, A. (1987) 'Bias in a survey of drinking habits', *Alcohol and Alcoholism*, Vol. 22, No. 2, pp. 167–79.

Department of Health (DoH) (1997) *The New NHS: Modern, Dependable*, London, HMSO.

Finkel, S., Guerbock, T. and Borg, M. (1991) 'Race-of-interviewer effects in a pre-election poll: Virginia 1989', *Public Opinion Quarterly*, Vol. 55, pp. 313–30.

Hall, J. and Dornan, M. (1988) 'Meta-analysis of satisfaction with medical care: description of research domain and analysis of overall satisfaction levels', *Social Science and Medicine*, Vol. 27, pp. 637–44.

Hall, J. and Dornan, M. (1990) 'Patient socio-demographic characteristics as predictors of satisfaction with medical care: a meta-analysis', *Social Science and Medicine*, Vol. 30, pp. 811–18.

Hamm, R., Hicks, R. and Bemben, D. (1996) 'Antibiotics and respiratory infections: are patients more satisfied when expectations are met?', *Journal of Family Practice*, Vol. 43, pp. 56–62.

Health Service Journal (1999) 'Shoddy league tables fall apart on the most cursory inspection', *Health Service Journal*, 17 June, p. 17.

Jenkinson, C. (ed.) (1994) *Measuring Health and Medical Outcomes*, London, UCL Press.

Kinsey, A., Pomeroy, W. and Martin, C. (1948) *Sexual Behaviour in the Human Male*, Philadelphia, W. B. Saunders.

Kinsey, A., Pomeroy, W., Martin, C. and Gebhard, P. (1953) *Sexual Behaviour in the Human Female*, Philadelphia, W. B. Saunders.

Lewis, G. and Wilkinson, G. (1993) 'Another British disease? A recent increase in the prevalence of psychiatric morbidity', *Journal of Epidemiology and Community Health*, Vol. 47, pp. 358–61.

Locker, D. and Dunt, D. (1978) 'Theoretical and mythological issues in sociological studies of consumer satisfaction with medical care', *Social Science and Medicine*, Vol. 12, pp. 283–92.

McIver, S. and Meredith, B. (1998) 'There for the asking', *Health Service Journal*, 19 February, pp. 26–27.

Meltzer, H., Gill, B., Petticrew, M. and Hinds, K. (1995) *The Prevalence of Psychiatric Morbidity Among Adults Living in Private Households: Report 1: OPCS Surveys of Psychiatric Morbidity in Great Britain*, London, HMSO.

Nathanson, C. (1978) 'Sex roles as variables in the interpretation of morbidity data: a methodological critique', *International Journal of Epidemiology*, Vol. 7, No. 3, pp. 253–62.

National Foundation for Mental Health (1995) *One in Four*, London, National Foundation for Mental Health.

National Health Service in Scotland (1993) *The Patient's Charter: What Users Think 1992*, Edinburgh, Scottish Office.

National Health Service in Scotland (1994) *The Patient's Charter: What Users Think 1993*, Edinburgh, Scottish Office.

Nazroo, J. (1997) *Mental Health and Ethnicity: Findings from a National Community Study*, London, Policy Studies Institute.

O'Connell-Davidson, J. and Layder, D. (1994) *Methods, Sex and Madness*, London, Routledge.

Packman, J., Randall, J. and Jacques, N. (1986) *Who Needs Care? Social Work Decisions About Children*, Oxford, Basil Blackwell.

Rudat, K. (1994) *Black and Minority Ethnic Groups in England: Health and Lifestyles*, London, Health Education Authority.

Savage, R. and Armstrong, D. (1990) 'Effect of a general practitioner's consulting style on patients' satisfaction: a controlled study', *British Medical Journal*, Vol. 301, pp. 968–70.

Stimson, G. and Webb, B. (1975) *Going To See the Doctor: The Consultation Process in General Practice*, London, Routledge and Kegan Paul.

Tudor-Smith, C., Nutbeam, D., Moore, L. and Catford, J. (1998) 'Effects of the Heartbeat Wales programme over five years on behavioural risks for cardiovascular disease: quasi-experimental comparison of results from Wales and a matched reference area', *British Medical Journal*, Vol. 316, pp. 818–22.

Wensing, M., Grol, R. and Smits, A. (1994) 'Quality judgements by patients on general practice care: a literature review', *Social Science and Medicine*, Vol. 38, pp. 45–53.

Williams, B. (1994) 'Patient satisfaction: a valid concept?', *Social Science and Medicine*, Vol. 38, pp. 509–16.

Chapter 3
Understanding experimental design

Roger Gomm

Introduction

Some people can inveigle their doctor into prescribing an antibiotic when they have influenza. Then, when they get better, as nearly all of them will, they attribute their cure to the antibiotic (Britten, 1995). And why not? The one thing followed the other.

There are two points to this example. The first is that people are constantly making incorrect causal attributions. This is not because they are foolish, but for two other kinds of reason. First, what is causing what is usually all mixed up with other things going on at the same time. Second, it is an ordinary human characteristic for people to perceive what they expect to perceive, and usually what they want to perceive. It takes a great deal of discipline to do otherwise. The second point of the example is that it can be said with great confidence that antibiotics will not cure viral infections. The two points are related. On the one hand, it is experimental research which provides this confidence. On the other hand, this confidence derives from the way an experimental approach can see through the interconnectedness of everything, and outflank the normal human tendency to discover what is familiar and congenial, rather than what is true.

This chapter looks at experimental approaches to producing evidence relevant to health and social care practice. First it considers *controlled experiments* which are what everyone thinks of when they hear the term 'experiment'. Among these are *randomised controlled* designs. In this chapter they are treated as an ideal against which other kinds of experiments appear as deficient. Later the chapter looks at *natural experiments*, where data collected from surveys or from agency records are analysed experimentally.

1 Experimental approaches

In a *controlled experiment* an artificial situation is created so that the multiple causes of phenomena can be controlled, by excluding some influences, standardising others, while allowing others to vary. This is called *controlling variables to prevent confounding*. 'Confounding' means muddling the picture so that it is difficult to discern what is causing what to happen (Campbell and Stanley, 1996).

Two basic designs

The two basic experimental designs are shown in Figure 1. The first answers questions about the effects of different interventions for similar people. It is the typical design used for trialling pharmaceuticals. The second answers questions about the different effects of the same intervention for different people. Here the question might be whether an intervention was equally effective for people from different ethnic groups. Sometimes the subjects are not people, or even parts of people, such as their hearts or eyes, but instruments, agencies or communities. Sometimes it is not treatments which are of interest but, for example, questionnaires (Chapter 2, Section 3), health education campaigns (Tudor-Smith *et al.*, 1998), or unplanned exposures to pathogens (Coggan *et al.*, 1993). It might be better to call the designs 'similar subjects/different *somethings*' and vice versa.

Surveys are not experiments as such, but surveys are different subjects/similar somethings designs. Chapter 2 noted the importance of always treating respondents to a survey as similarly as possible.

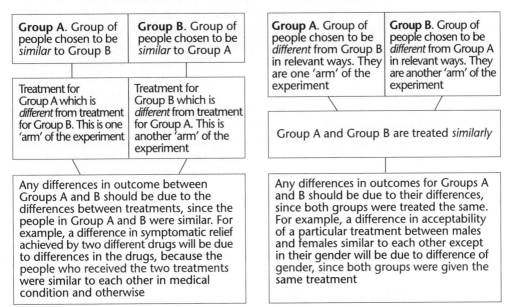

Figure 1 **Two basic experimental designs: (a) a similar subjects/different treatments design; (b) a different subjects/similar treatments design**

Starting at the end and working backwards

As with surveys (Chapter 2, Section 1), experimenters are looking for statistically significant differences. In a similar subjects/different treatments design, any statistically significant differences recorded between the groups of subjects at the end of the experiment should demonstrate the effects of intentional differences in the way they were treated: the so-called *treatment* or *intervention effect*. If the question is 'What makes the results of an experiment believable?', the answer is in terms of how well the researcher has managed to exclude things other than the intended differences in treatment from influencing the results. To a large extent, saying that the results of an experiment are (internally) valid is saying that unwanted influences on the results of the experiment have been excluded or *controlled*. The means of exclusion are listed as 'safeguards' in Table 1 (opposite and overleaf).

Experiments as systems of safeguards

The term 'safeguards' is used advisedly. Randomised controlled trials (which are described in Section 2) have developed over the last 50 years as a means of preventing any preconceptions, desires and sloppiness on behalf of experimenters from producing erroneous results (Cochrane, 1972). There are many examples of dangerous and ineffectual practices being foisted on the public because of inadequate experimental work, although these are probably greatly outnumbered by dangerous and ineffective interventions that have not been tested experimentally at all (Oakley, 1989). The safeguards indicated will not necessarily protect against determined cheats. They usually get caught out when someone repeats or *replicates* their research (British Medical Journal, 1998). Experimental research is often replicated. This means, first, that rogue results become apparent in a series of experiments on the same topic and, second, that the results of several small-scale experiments can be combined to produce composite findings in which practitioners can have more confidence (see Chapter 7).

The safeguards shown in Table 1 will go a long way to preventing researchers or practitioners being misled by their own preferences for achieving one result rather than another. For readers of research, the 'safeguards' are pointers to questions they might ask in appraising research.

Table 1 **Sources of confounding in experiments and safeguards against them**

Statistically significant differences in outcome may be due to the differences caused by the intended intervention, but they might also be due in part or in whole to any of the factors in the left-hand column below, if the safeguards in the right-hand column have not been used.

Causes of *differences* in outcomes between the arms of the experiment other than the intended differences in treatment	Safeguards that might prevent such factors confounding the results
1 Prior differences between the comparison groups (see also 2)	Use the best means available for creating comparison groups: preferably randomisation. Cross-check that groups are near-equivalent at the outset (Section 2)
2 Differences between groups emerging because of differential pattern of drop-out or swap-over or experimental expectation	Prevent practitioners knowing which group subjects have been allocated to – known as 'blinding' – to prevent bias influencing drop-out or swap-over. Report results in terms of treatment subjects were supposed to receive, even if they did not – reporting in terms of intention to treat. (Section 3) Check that groups are near-equivalent at end of experiment
3 Differences between groups emerging because subjects know which group they are in so that this knowledge influences their behaviour or response to treatment in a way that should be irrelevant to the experiment	Prevent subjects knowing which treatment they are getting – known as 'blinding' (Section 3)
4 One group having more extreme scores at the outset than another and hence showing more 'improvement' due to regression to the mean	As for 1 and analyse statistically to estimate for possibility of regression effect (Section 4)
5 Differences between groups arising because of differential rates of non-compliance between subjects in different arms of the trial	Monitor subject compliance. Report results in terms of the treatment subjects were supposed to receive, even if they did not – reporting in terms of intention to treat (Section 3)
6 Differences between groups arising because of *unintended* differences in treatment, differences of practitioner expertise, and so on	Devise and monitor protocol for way subjects should be treated. Allocate same practitioners equally to all arms. In so far as unintended differences of treatment are due to practitioner bias, blind practitioners about treatment subjects are receiving (Section 3)

(*continued*)

Table 1 (*continued*)

7 Differences due to bias in assessment/measurement	Prevent those who are assessing/measuring knowing which arm of a trial subjects are in – blinding. For example, use blinded, independent judges (Section 3)
8 Differences between groups arising because of extraneous factors influencing one group more than another	This may be difficult to control or estimate where many factors might influence results and subjects are often out of view of experimenters. Devices such as subject diaries or interviews might help. A large sample will give a better chance of such factors balancing out across all arms of the trial and/or will reduce the influence of rare events on the results

No statistically significant difference in outcome in the results may be due to there being no difference in effect between the treatments in the trial, or between intervention and non-intervention, **but might be due** to any of the factors in the left-hand column below if the safeguards in the right-hand column have not been used.

Causes of *similarity* of outcome between arms of a trial, other than similarity of effect of different treatments or of treatment and non-intervention	Safeguards that might prevent such factors confounding the results
9 *Unintended* similarities of treatment	Devise and monitor protocol for way subjects should be treated. In so far as unintended similarity arose from biases of practitioners, prevent practitioners knowing group membership of subjects (Section 3)
10 Non-compliance by subjects in treatment arm of a trial so that many of them did not actually receive the treatment	Monitor subject compliance (also see 5)
11 Ineffectual blinding of subjects where an experiment relies on blinding – as in many psychological experiments	Effective blinding of subjects (Section 3)
12 Subjects in all arms of the trial having extreme scores at the outset so that any treatment differences are submerged by the effects of regression to the mean	Avoid selecting a group of subjects with an extreme average score. Analyse statistically to estimate regression effect (Senn, 1997)
13 Sample too small to allow for detection of real differences in effect between intended treatments	Use adequately sized sample (Altman, 1991, pp. 455–60)
14 Use of measurement instrument too insensitive to small differences or too over-sensitive to irrelevant differences	Use appropriate measurement instrument (Jenkinson, 1994)

2 Randomised controlled trials

Randomised controlled experiments or trials (RCTs) use the strongest set of safeguards against the troubles indicated above (see Table 1). The properly conducted, correctly interpreted RCT is superior to any other method for producing evidence about cause and effect. This includes evidence about the effectiveness of health and social care interventions (Shepperd *et al.*, 1997). Where other methods depart from the RCT format, they usually produce evidence about cause and effect of a lower quality. Thus what follows below is a discussion of RCTs as an ideal against which other kinds of research into causality can be judged.

Randomisation

The most distinctive feature of an RCT is that the comparison groups of subjects are created *at random* (Roberts and Sibbald, 1998). Methods range from tossing coins to using a computer program. As with probability sampling in surveys, the principle is that each subject entering the experiment should have an equal chance of being allocated to any of the different treatments: that is, to any of the 'arms' of the trial (see Figure 1). Each group of subjects should be a representative sample of all the subjects involved. Randomisation maximises the chances that any prior differences between subjects will crop up in equal proportions in each arm of the trial, thus balancing each other out. This is to avoid such differences contaminating the results. This can be cross-checked in terms of knowable characteristics, such as age, gender, body weight, and so on at the beginning and at the end of the trial.

Methods other than randomisation are used in other experimental designs – for example, a 'matched pairs' strategy may be used, sorting subjects into pairs similar to each other on a number of criteria (Bowling, 1997, pp. 220–22). One of each pair is allocated to each treatment. This last is often done at random but it would not make such an experiment a randomised controlled trial. The term 'quasi-randomisation' might be used. Creating comparison groups like this relies on characteristics that are identifiable. It may disproportionately allocate important factors which are unknown, invisible or overlooked. It would be possible to divide a pack of cards into two groups, each precisely similar in terms of numbers of reds and blacks, numbers of picture cards, and so on. But that might still result in most of the dog-eared cards being in one of the two piles. Since the important characteristics of the subjects may be unknown at the outset (and often afterwards too), randomisation is preferred, even though it may not allocate visible characteristics between groups so precisely as other methods would. Schultz and his colleagues (1995) have investigated the effects of different designs on the outcomes of research. They suggest that even in randomised controlled trials, slipshod randomisation may result in spurious differences of up to 40% of the outcome differences shown. When comparison groups are created by means other than randomisation, results are likely, and spuriously, to show greater outcome differences than would have been the case in an RCT. This will be due to uncontrolled prior differences between the groups seeping through to the results.

3   Blinding to control subject reactions and professional misjudgements

Rosenthal and Rubin's (1978) classic experiments about experiments in the 1970s demonstrated that even laboratory rats behave more intelligently if experimenters are led to believe that they are more intelligent rats and, similarly, that the behaviour of human subjects in experiments is strongly influenced by what experimenters expect to happen. Again the whole weight of psychological research suggests that unwittingly biased judgements by researchers are more likely than unbiased ones if no means are taken to prevent this (Sadler, 1981). The term *blinding* refers to preventing subjects, practitioners and/or experimenters knowing something where that knowledge might influence the results of the experiment in a way it should not do (Pocock, 1983).

The classic blind involves the use of *placebo* treatments. For example, a dose of vitamin C may be made up to look and taste like the pharmaceutical being tested and the two administered in such a way that the subjects, the practitioners and the experimenters do not at the time know which is which.

Table 2 distinguishes some different kinds of blinding.

In some circumstances, effective blinding may not be possible and other strategies may be adopted as a fall-back position. Blinding practitioners as to which of the treatments subjects are receiving is rarely practicable in surgery, social work, counselling or health education. For assessing effects many RCTs instead use independent judges who are blinded as to which treatments subjects have received.

Intention to treat

Without blinding, the biases of practitioners or experimenters may influence the make-up of the comparison groups through influencing who drops out. To safeguard against this, it is common to report results for all subjects whether they dropped out or not and in terms of *intention to treat* (Shepperd *et al.*, 1997, pp. 11–12). Here the results for subjects are reported according to the treatment they were supposed to receive even if they have swapped to another arm or are behaving like members of another arm of the trial. Reporting in terms of intention to treat is the next line of defence if blinding is not appropriate, or if it is ineffectual.

Table 2   Blinding and the problems of not blinding

	With unblinded subjects	With unblinded practitioners	With unblinded researchers
Blind allocation to comparison groups (this is usually accomplished automatically by random allocation)	Comparison groups may differ from each other in ways associated with different kinds of subjects making choices of group membership	Comparison groups may differ from each other in ways arising from the preferences of practitioners influencing the way subjects are allocated to groups	Comparison groups may differ from each other in ways arising from the biases of the researcher influencing the way subjects are allocated to groups
Blind to treatment being received (for example, by using a placebo, or by making two treatments look identical)	Subjects' responses to the treatment may be influenced by their knowledge of the treatment they are getting	Practitioners may treat subjects in different arms of the trial differently in ways they should not, because they believe in one treatment more than another	Researchers' perceptions of what happens may be biased by their knowledge of which treatment is being given
Blind to treatment received	Follow-up investigations of subjects' perceptions of their experience during the research may be influenced by knowing which treatment they received	Practitioners' judgements of outcomes may be biased by knowing which treatment subjects received	Researchers' judgements of outcomes may be biased by knowing which treatment subjects received

Failing that, researchers should at least provide an account of the characteristics of those who dropped out in comparison with those who did not. This is to see whether different kinds of people dropped out of each arm, thus causing the groups to be dissimilar and producing differences in the results attributable to this. This is the same principle as for the analysis of the non-response in a survey (Chapter 2, Section 2).

Experiment effects

Blinding prevents bias influencing the outcomes in one arm of a trial more than in another and hence producing spurious outcome differences. But it is also possible that simply knowing that they are involved in an experiment will influence people's responses. This may happen irrespective of which arm of the trial they are allocated to or whether they know which. This is sometimes called an *experiment* or a *reactive effect* (Bowling,

1997, p. 137). It may or may not create outcome differences between arms of the trial. But it may create results that will not transfer to routine practice, since in routine practice clients' interpretations of what is going on will be different from those of people who know they are subjects in an experiment.

4   Generalising from experimental results

The internal validity of an experiment is the extent to which any differences or similarities shown on an outcome measure are due to the intended treatments given *and not to anything else*. RCTs in particular can achieve very high levels of internal validity (Section 1) because of the strong control exerted over variables. *External validity*, however, is a synonym for *generalisability*, which refers to the extent that what was true in the research will be true and meaningful for other people in other places.

Research that is internally *in*valid cannot be generalised. But even if research is internally valid it may not be generalisable, or it may only be generalisable to situations that would occur only rarely in real life. Here the artificiality of the experiment can be a problem when attempts are made to transfer research findings into practice (Black, 1996; Altman and Bland, 1998).

For example, it is common in medical trials to reduce the need for a large sample size by starting out with a pool of subjects which is very homogeneous. Many such trials are single sex, with subjects from a narrow age-span and exclude patients with 'complications'. Thus nearly all RCTs on treatments for hypertension have been conducted on people who suffer from hypertension and nothing else. But in practice 90% of patients presenting with hypertension have at least one other serious medical condition as well (Tudor-Hart, 1993). Since few RCTs begin with random samples drawn from a known population, most rate rather low for *representativeness*. Usually, randomised controlled trials begin with a *convenience* or *grab* sample: just those people who happen to be around when a sample is needed, then whittled down by excluding those who have problems that would complicate the experiment, or who are too sick or refuse to participate. Thus the randomisation which creates comparison groups in an RCT will make each group a representative sample of all subjects entering the experiment, but only rarely will all subjects together be a representative sample drawn from a known population (see Chapter 2, Section 2).

However, it is important not to assume that difficulty of generalisation is only associated with RCTs. A study conducted under the ordinary, workaday circumstances of a children's home will also produce results which are difficult to generalise to another children's home where ordinary, workaday conditions are likely to be different (see Chapter 9). Here, if anything, the problem of generalisation may be worse. The artificiality of experimental conditions is compensated for, somewhat, to the extent that these conditions are clearly specified. Then judgements can be made about how like or unlike are the circumstances of the experiment and the circumstance of practice. Specification of this kind is easier in experimental research, where variables are identified and controlled, than it is in more naturalistic settings for research (see Chapters 4 and 5).

Applying experimental research findings in practice is dealt with in more detail in Chapters 7 to 10, but among the difficulties is that of applying information about groups to the design of interventions for individuals.

From group means to individualised treatments

Typically, RCTs and other controlled experiments report their results in terms of scores for groups. A group score showing an effective intervention may clump together people who made huge improvements with people who did not and perhaps with people who actually got worse. Some trials report 'indications' and 'contra-indications' but many do not. Then the only practical reading of the results will be in terms of what to do in order to effect the greatest amount of benefit for the greatest number of people, while knowing that this will mean subjecting some people to treatments from which they will derive no benefit and might suffer some harm (Jelinek, 1992; Nutting and Green, 1994). What is needed is some way of bridging the gap between results for groups and predictions for individual clients. Experiments large enough to distinguish sub-groups for separate statistical analysis is one possibility. But this is extremely expensive.

Another way is to extend experimentalism into practice. The individualised version of the RCT is the *n-of-1 experiment* (Campbell, 1994). These usually start from the results of a group trial, but now there is only one subject for the experiment – the client, who acts as both experimental subject and control in turn. Two treatments, or an active treatment and a placebo, are given to the client one after another in random sequence, with both the practitioner and the client blind to the treatment being given. Outcomes are recorded. After several swaps it usually becomes quite clear that neither or one or the other is more effective. At that stage the experiment ends. The blinding is undone, and clinician and client know which is the more effective of the two, or that neither of them works (Shepperd *et al.*, 1997, pp. 17–18).

Unfortunately, n-of-1 trials can only be conducted with treatments that do not have long-lasting effects, because this would extend the effect of one treatment into the period when another was being given. Pain control is a common area for n-of-1 experiments. What makes the n-of-1 trial particularly convincing is the blinding. In practice, practitioners often do something rather like n-of-1 experiments without blinding when they seek to stabilise a drug regime for a patient, or pin down a source of food allergy by systematically excluding items from the diet.

In clinical psychology and social work the analogue of n-of-1 trials is *single-case*, or *single-system*, evaluation (Kazi and Wilson, 1996; Bloom, 1993). Again there is only one subject for the experiment. Blinding is not appropriate since the client and practitioner have to know which intervention is being given. Since randomisation in the n-of-1 is only used as a blind, randomisation is not used here either. Thus the experiment consists of alternating a period of intervention with a period of non-intervention, or alternating two interventions. For example, in treating childhood enuresis a period of fulsome praise for a dry bed may be alternated with a period when dry beds are treated as normal and nothing to make a fuss about. Some children respond better to the one; some to the other. On an outcome measure of nights without bed-wetting this should show either that neither treatment is effective, or that one is more effective than the other. In the latter case a ratchet effect is to be expected, with the deterioration in each succeeding period of the less effective treatment never falling back so far as recorded in the previous period of less effective treatment.

These kinds of experimentation are often consistent with routine practice and if published may help to fill in the details about 'what exactly works for whom', which is often left unexamined in group experiments.

5   Quasi-experiments and natural experiments

Quasi-experiments are variations on the basic designs shown in Figure 1, but use means other than randomisation for creating comparison groups (Campbell and Stanley, 1966). One way of reading accounts of quasi-experiments is to look for the ways in which their design departs from a blinded RCT and deduct points for credibility accordingly. For example, Tudor-Smith and his colleagues (1998) attempted to evaluate the effectiveness of the large-scale *Heartbeat Wales* health education programme, using a pre-intervention and a post-intervention survey in Wales, and, for comparison, in an area in North East England. The survey gathered data about behaviours relevant to coronary heart disease. This is a *reference group* or *reference area* design. The example illustrates the problem that arises when experimenters have no control over what happens to the control group. Here the role of the control group was played by the reference area in the North East. While people in North East England had not been influenced by *Heartbeat Wales*, they had been bombarded with health education messages from other sources. Since both areas showed improvements in health-related behaviours it was impossible to demonstrate whether *Heartbeat Wales* had any effect at all.

Again so-called 'pre/post test studies without controls' merely compare the same subjects before and after the same treatment. They have no credibility at all in judging the effectiveness of an intervention, except to the extent that they can be bench-marked on research or practice elsewhere. For example, in clinical audit the local team may derive pre/ post test data for their own clients and compare these with published data from other areas (Firth-Cozens, 1993, p. 9). Many performance indicators in health and social care are used for bench-marking in this way. The data from elsewhere then provide an external comparison which in a full-blown experimental design would be built into the experimental structure. But making external comparisons like this runs the risk of comparing unlike with unlike. Perhaps the subjects elsewhere were not quite like those here. Perhaps what they did elsewhere was not quite like what was done locally.

However, a well-conducted quasi-experiment may deserve more confidence than a badly conducted RCT. Any experiment of any kind can founder due to unreliability (see Chapter 2, Section 3): for example, those subjects who should be treated alike not being treated alike; those who should be treated differently being treated similarly; differences of practitioner expertise contaminating the results; subjects, unbeknown to the researcher, not complying with their treatments, and so on.

Natural experiments

In many situations it would be unethical or impractical to use a controlled experiment but a *natural experiment* can be used instead. The term 'natural experiment' is used to refer to the experimentalist *analysis* of data about events which happen without being created for research purposes. The study of children being resettled from Eastern European orphanages is a recent example in the field of child development studies (Rutter, 1999). However, more usually, the data are those collected by surveys or through routine bureaucratic procedures such as agency record-keeping or official certification (Procter, 1993). The *Heartbeat Wales* example above was a social survey. It is described by its authors as a quasi-experiment but it differs only from natural experiments in so far as the health education programme was a deliberate intervention. Otherwise its approach is very similar, and presents the same problems.

Control over variables is not achieved here by creating an artificial environment. Instead data about naturally occurring events are controlled statistically. The data are sifted into different categories in an attempt to make the subjects in each category identical in all respects except one. For example, if white males and African-Caribbean males of the *same* social class had *different* rates of psychoses diagnosed then it would seem as if ethnicity rather than social class were the important factor. Or if ethnic differences in rates of diagnosed psychoses were lower when analysed by social class, the reduction in difference could be taken as a measure of the influence of social class on psychosis, independently of ethnicity. Just as in an experiment proper, here two variables – social class and ethnicity –

would have been controlled (Nazroo, 1997): although the control would certainly be weaker than in a controlled experiment. The age-weighting featured in Table 1 of Chapter 2 is another example of statistical control.

Natural experiments may be used for studying the effectiveness of interventions or policies. This is typical, for example, in the study of the effects of educational policies. But they are much more commonly used for investigating the causes of illness, or antecedents of social or behavioural problems. This is in order to specify high-risk groups, or identify points at which interventions might be made for preventative work (Barker and Rose, 1990; Rutter, 1994; Macdonald, 1994).

The quality of findings from a natural experiment depends on the quality of the data used. Bureaucratically collected data, such as on death certificates, often leaves much to be desired (Sapsford and Abbott, 1992, pp. 64–65; Bloor et al., 1987). Quite competently collected survey data may not have been collected for the purpose of the analysis to which a researcher wants to subject it. The critical questions may not have been asked or the kinds of people of interest may make up only a small percentage of the sample.

Retrospective and prospective studies

Many surveys and many bureaucratic data sets are 'cross-sectional': recording data at a single point in time thus allowing only for *retrospective* study (Mant and Jenkinson, 1997). These kinds of data indicate what is associated with what (correlations) rather than what preceded what. It is from the latter that what caused what may be more confidently inferred. Thus, for example, correlations between unemployment and early death might mean that unemployment was part of the cause of premature mortality. But it might mean that the people more likely to die sooner were sicker and more likely than others to lose their jobs. This *direction of effect* problem is common in the analysis of cross-sectional data.

In *prospective* studies, data are collected *before* the events of interest have happened, just as in a controlled experiment. Not only are data collected about the same people at different time points, but the data are preserved against forgetting, and from the effects of *retrospective bias* which happens as people reconstruct their memories in the light of what has happened subsequently (Mant and Jenkinson, 1997). Practitioners and researchers are just as prone to this form of bias as are clients. Prospective studies accomplish a kind of blinding (Section 3) because people supply and record information while blind to the significance it might have in a future analysis.

The best-known prospective studies are the national child development studies: variously called longitudinal surveys, cohort studies or panel studies. These survey all, or a large sample, of the children born during one week in 1946, 1958 and 1970 throughout their lives. They have the advantage of being representative samples of all kinds of children born in the UK at the time of their birth (except with regard to children born at different times of year). These studies constitute an invaluable bank of knowledge about child and, now, adult development for child care and child health practice (Wadsworth, 1991). But comprehensiveness can be at the cost of not capturing enough of some kinds of children for some kinds of investigation: again the problem of sub-groups being too small for analytic purposes. Drop-out, which is the characteristic non-response feature of a longitudinal survey, is a problem. It is easier to manage than in a retrospective study, since much is already known about those who drop out from data already collected about them. A particular problem with birth cohort studies is that they take a very long time. The people in the 1946 birth cohort were only 54 years old in the year 2000. It will be 2015 before it will be clear what effect early childhood experience in the 1940s had on health and welfare in old age. The circumstances in which these children grew up will then be long gone. Although the results of these studies might be generalisable to the whole British-born population of similar age, much will be difficult to generalise to subsequent generations.

More sharply focused and/or shorter duration cohort studies are often used. For example, there is the longitudinal study of mortality from 1971 onwards (Goldblatt, 1990). This is an important source of data on the causal relationships between illness, work, premature death and social class. In child development there is a long tradition running from earlier studies such as those comparing a cohort of children on the Isle of Wight with another in an inner London Borough (Rutter *et al.*, 1975a and b), or the Newsons' well-known studies of child-bearing and child-rearing in Nottingham (for example, Newson and Newson, 1963), or West and Farrington's study of the development of delinquency (1973), to the more recent Avon Longitudinal Study of Pregnancy and Childhood (Dunn, 1999). A landmark cohort study in medicine was that investigating the relationship between heart disease, lung cancer and smoking, by Doll and Hill (1964), using a cohort of doctors (68% of all doctors in 1951), dividing them into whether they were smokers or non-smokers at the time and then tracing their cause of death through death certification until 1961.

6   Case control studies

Case control studies sit between controlled experiments and natural experiments (Mant and Jenkinson, 1997). They are like natural experiments in so far as the 'cases' arise naturally. They usually feature cases cropping up in practice. And they are like controlled experiments in so far as the experimenter goes out and finds some real people to be controls. Thus Burton *et al.* (1998) started with cases of children who had experienced homelessness. They then found a group of children with a similar age, gender, social class and ethnic mix who had not experienced homelessness, and compared the physical and mental health of the two groups. This is a retrospective case control design because what was studied had already happened. Prospective versions are also possible. For example, Heath and his colleagues (1994) used a cohort of children in foster care (the cases) and a cohort of children from similar backgrounds but living with their own families (the controls). They argued that, since previous research had shown very little difference between children cared for by social services and those 'known to' social services, this was a good matching (Campbell, 1991). Then they followed the educational development of the two groups over three years. The results demonstrated the ineffectiveness of social services in promoting educational achievement among the children in their care.

Case control studies are popular. The method can be used where it would often be unethical or impractical to do a controlled experiment on the one hand, and where, on the other, using the natural experimental method might require a large-scale survey, or where there are no appropriate existing data sets for the topic at hand. Unfortunately, case control studies tend to combine the weaknesses of these approaches (Mant and Jenkinson, 1997). First, the method of creating controls which are truly similar to the cases falls far short of what can be achieved by randomisation. Convenience tends to loom large in many studies. There are always grave risks that any differences shown between groups are artefacts created by the methods of recruiting controls, rather than differences associated with the critical variable. Second, where they are retrospective studies, as with all retrospective studies, they are beset with problems about whether associations between variables indicate causal links or not, and with problems of retrospective bias. Third, they are very vulnerable to confounding in ways related to processes through which cases come to be known about: *ascertainment bias* (Mant and Jenkinson, 1997, p. 35). Thus a case control study of child abuse might show some family differences between the cases of abused children and the controls who were not abused. This might indicate something about the cause of child abuse. Alternatively, it might indicate something about the causes of child abuse being detected or not.

What are sometimes called *case finding studies* have no controls as such. Rather, cases known about are simply compared with what is known about the general population from which they were drawn. The results of a case control study usually deserve more confidence than the results of a case finding study.

Conclusion

Some people find experimental approaches constricting. Some faced with all the 'ifs and buts' raised by experimentalism look elsewhere for a less problematic alternative. However, on the first count, experimentalism is *supposed* to be constricting. It is supposed to discipline thought so that people do not make unwarranted assumptions about what causes what or about which interventions are effective ones. All the safeguards against bias associated with an experimentalist approach may make it seem as if people cannot be trusted to make unbiased judgements. But research has demonstrated that without such safeguards this is actually so.

On the second count, the ifs and buts, caveats and provisos that surround any experimental study are a mark of strength rather than of weakness. All kinds of research raise similar difficulties where issues of causality and generalisability are concerned. But experimental research is designed to make these problems visible, and hence manageable. In other kinds of research, these problems may remain invisible, unmanageable and misleading.

This chapter also illustrates again that different methods of research have different strengths and different weaknesses. Consider, for example, the topic of consumer satisfaction. The satisfaction surveys featured in Chapter 2 were based on well conducted survey research using large representative samples. With some caveats, it was possible to say with confidence that the patterns of responses from those surveyed represented the pattern that would have been recorded had everyone in the population been asked the same questions in the same way. But neither survey provides much information about what actually happened to these patients to provoke them to give the responses they gave, or whether, indeed, their satisfactions and dissatisfactions were caused by their encounters with health services.

Thus a high level of generalisability was accompanied by a weakness in demonstrating cause and effect. This was one reason why it was suggested that such data are of limited used for performance monitoring. Savage and Armstrong (1990) conducted a randomised controlled experiment in general practice in which patients received one of two styles of communication from the GP: either a highly directive style or a more sharing and facilitative one. In a follow-up at two weeks, the patients who had received the more directive style expressed themselves as being much more satisfied than the others in various ways. In this case it is possible to attribute the satisfaction scores directly to the differences in communication styles experienced. The experimental design eliminated other possibilities (see Table 1). However, this experiment was conducted in one, inner-urban, multi-ethnic practice, which is not representative of all practices, and may not even be representative of all inner-urban, multi-ethnic ones. Thus, although experimentally sound, the results of the experiment cannot be generalised to other practices with any confidence.

Neither approaches to 'satisfaction' get very close to the clients' experiences of being satisfied or not, or any other aspect of their experience. For that purpose, another style of research is required. That is the subject of the next chapter. When reading it, it is important to realise that the more we concentrate on the unique meanings of events to people, the less we are able to generalise about these, and the less we learn about the causes of what happens to them. We would not learn what cured influenza by studying the medical beliefs of the patients at the start of this chapter who asked their doctors for antibiotics. But by doing so we might learn some other interesting things about them.

References

Altman, D. (1991) *Practical Statistics for Medical Research*, London, Chapman and Hall.

Altman, D. and Bland, J. (1998) 'Generalisation and extrapolation', *British Medical Journal*, Vol. 317, pp. 409–10.

Barker, D. and Rose, G. (1990) *Epidemiology in Medical Practice*, Edinburgh, Churchill Livingstone.

Black, N. (1996) 'Why we need observational studies to evaluate the effectiveness of health care', *British Medical Journal*, Vol. 312, pp. 1215–18.

Bloom, M. (1993) (ed.) *Single-system Designs in the Social Services: Issues and Options for the 1990s*, New York, Haworth.

Bloor, M., Samphier, M. and Prior, L. (1987) 'Artefact explanations of inequalities in health: an assessment of the evidence', *Sociology of Health and Illness*, Vol. 9, No. 3, pp. 231–64.

Bowling, A. (1997) *Research Methods in Health: Investigating Health and Health Services*, Buckingham, Open University Press.

British Medical Journal (1998) Section devoted to research misconduct, *British Medical Journal*, Vol. 316, pp. 1726–33.

Britten, N. (1995) 'Patients' ideas about medicine: a qualitative study in a general practice population', *British Journal of General Practice*, Vol. 44, pp. 465–68.

Burton, G., Blair, M. and Crown, N. (1998) 'A new look at the health and homeless experience of a cohort of five-year-olds', *Children and Society*, Vol. 12, pp. 349–58.

Campbell, M. (1991) 'Children at risk: how different are children on child abuse registers?', *British Journal of Social Work*, Vol. 21, pp. 259–75.

Campbell, M. (1994) 'Commentary: *n* of 1 trials may be useful for informed decision making', *British Medical Journal*, Vol. 309, pp. 1044–45.

Campbell, T. and Stanley, J. (1996) *Experimental and Quasi-experimental Designs for Research*, Chicago, Rand McNally.

Cochrane, A. (1972) *Effectiveness and Efficiency*, Oxford, Nuffield Provincial Hospitals Trust.

Coggan, D., Rose, G. and Barker, D. (1993) *Epidemiology for the Uninitiated*, London, BMJ Publications.

Doll, R. and Hill, A. (1964) 'Mortality in relation to smoking: ten years' observation of British doctors', *British Medical Journal*, June, pp. 1399–1410 and pp. 1460–67.

Dunn, J. (1999) 'Happy families step by step', *Medical Research Council News*, No. 80, pp. 16–19.

Firth-Cozens, J. (1993) *Audit in Mental Health Services*, Hove, Lawrence Erlbaum Associates.

Goldblatt, P. (1990) (ed.) *Longitudinal Study: Mortality and Social Organisation 1971–81*, OPCS Series LS, No. 6, London, HMSO.

Heath, A., Colton, M. and Aldgate, J. (1994) 'Failure to escape: a longitudinal study of foster children's educational attainment', *British Journal of Social Work*, Vol. 24, pp. 241–60.

Jelinek, M. (1992) 'The clinician and the randomised controlled trial', in Daly, J., McDonald, I. and Willis, E. (eds) *Researching Health Care: Designs, Dilemmas, Disciplines*, pp. 76–90, London, Routledge.

Jenkinson, C. (1994) (ed.) *Measuring Health and Medical Outcomes*, London, UCL Press.

Kazi, M. and Wilson, J. (1996) 'Applying single-case evaluation in social work', *British Journal of Social Work*, Vol. 26, pp. 699–717.

Macdonald, G. (1994) 'Developing empirically-based practice in probation', *British Journal of Social Work*, Vol. 24, pp. 405–27.

Mant, J. and Jenkinson, C. (1997) 'Case control and cohort studies', in Jenkinson, C. (ed.) *Assessment and Evaluation of Health and Medical Care: A Methods Text*, pp. 31–46, Buckingham, Open University Press.

Nazroo, J. (1997) *Mental Health and Ethnicity: Findings from a National Community Survey*, London, Policy Studies Institute.

Newson, J. and Newson, E. (1963) *Infant Care in an Urban Community*, London, Allen and Unwin.

Nutting, P. and Green, L. (1994) 'From research to policy to practice: closing the loop in clinical policy development for primary care', in Dunn, E., Norton, P., Stewart, M., Tudover, F. and Bass, M. (eds) *Disseminating Research/Changing Practice*, pp. 151–61, London, Sage.

Oakley, A. (1989) 'Who's afraid of the randomised controlled trial? Some dilemmas of the scientific method and good research practice', *Women and Health*, Vol. 15, pp. 25–59.

Pocock, S. (1983) *Clinical Trials: A Practical Approach*, Englewood Cliffs, NJ, Prentice Hall.

Procter, M. (1993) 'Analysing survey data', in Gilbert, N. (ed.) *Researching Social Life*, pp. 239–54, London, Sage.

Roberts, C. and Sibbald, B. (1998) 'Randomising groups of patients', *British Medical Journal*, Vol. 316, p. 1898.

Rosenthal, R. and Rubin, D. (1978) 'Interpersonal expectancy effects: the first 345 studies', *The Behavioural and Brain Sciences*, Vol. 3, pp. 377–415.

Rutter, M. (1994) 'Beyond longitudinal data: causes, consequences, changes and continuity', *Journal of Consulting and Clinical Psychology*, Vol. 65, No. 5, pp. 928–40.

Rutter, M. (1999) 'Natural experiments to study psychosocial risk', *Medical Research Council News*, No. 80, pp. 24–27.

Rutter, M., Cox, A., Tupling, C., Berger, M. and Yule, W. (1975a) 'Attainment and adjustment in two geographical areas I: the prevalence of psychiatric disorder', *British Journal of Psychiatry*, Vol. 126, pp. 493–509.

Rutter, M., Yule, B., Morton, J. and Bagley, C. (1975b) 'Attainment and adjustment in two geographical areas III: some factors accounting for area differences', *British Journal of Psychiatry*, Vol. 126, pp. 520–33.

Sadler, D. R. (1981) 'Intuitive data processing as a potential source of bias in naturalistic evaluations', *Educational Evaluation and Policy Analysis*, July–August, pp. 25–31.

Sapsford, R. and Abbott, P. (1992) *Research Methods for Nurses and the Caring Professions*, Buckingham, Open University Press.

Savage, R. and Armstrong, D. (1990) 'Effect of a general practitioner's consulting style on patients' satisfaction: a controlled study', *British Medical Journal*, Vol. 301, pp. 968–70.

Schultz, K., Chalmers, I., Hayes, R. and Altman, D. (1995) 'Empirical evidence of bias: dimensions of methodological quality associated with estimates of treatment effects in controlled trials', *Journal of American Medical Association*, Vol. 273, pp. 408–12.

Senn, S. (1997) 'Regression to the mean', *Statistical Methods in Medical Research*, Vol. 6, pp. 99–102.

Shepperd, S., Doll, H. and Jenkinson, C. (1997) 'Randomized controlled trials', in Jenkinson, C. (ed.) *Assessment and Evaluation of Health and Medical Care: A Methods Text*, pp. 6–30, Buckingham, Open University Press.

Tudor-Hart, J. (1993) 'Hypertension guidelines: other diseases complicate management', *British Medical Journal*, Vol. 306, p. 1337.

Tudor-Smith, C., Nutbeam, D., Moore, L. and Catford, J. (1998) 'Effects of Heartbeat Wales programme over five years on behavioural risks for cardiovascular disease: quasi-experimental comparison of results from Wales and a matched reference area', *British Medical Journal*, Vol. 316, pp. 818–22.

Wadsworth, M. (1991) *The Imprint of Time: Childhood History and Adult Life*, Oxford, Clarendon.

West, D. and Farrington, D. (1973) *Who Becomes Delinquent?*, London, Heinemann.

Chapter 4
Interpreting meanings

Kelley Johnson

Introduction

Social interactions and relationships in everyday life are based on people understanding and interpreting the meanings and experiences others convey through their language or behaviour or those we construct together. Understanding and interpretation are also key concepts for many professionals working in health and social welfare whose skills include listening, questioning (both themselves and others), observing, empathising and analysing, in order to understand the needs and the requirements of clients or patients.

This approach to understanding the world and other people has been further reflected, distilled and 'fine tuned' in a range of different research approaches which can be described loosely as 'qualitative research'. Such research is quite different from the approach described in Chapter 3 in terms of experimental design, which looks for causal relations between variables, to be explained, predicted and to some extent controlled and which are assumed to exist independently of the researcher.

This chapter is concerned with how researchers have sought to understand and to interpret the meanings people give to issues affecting their lives or to their 'lived experience'. More particularly, the aims are:

- To introduce the diverse, and often hotly contested, ways in which qualitative research has been conceptualised by researchers.

- To examine the methods for collecting data in qualitative research as an exploration of meanings rather than a discovery of 'facts' or relationships between specific variables.

- To explore the explicit positioning of the researcher in qualitative research and the use of reflection as a methodological tool.

- To provide guidelines for assessing the quality and potential relevance of research findings, and research methods, to practice.

With these aims in mind, this chapter is largely framed as a personal exploration of the field of qualitative research and so is written in the first person.

1   Two contrasting case studies

Over time, and in different contexts, researchers adopt different ways of finding answers to questions which trouble, vex or obsess them (see Denzin and Lincoln, 1998). This section describes briefly two research projects in which I have been involved, one at the beginning of my life as a researcher, the other more recently. Each in its own way was concerned with how people construct meanings. Both were also concerned with how an increased understanding of these meanings might lead to changes in behaviour, professional practices and societal change. However, they demonstrate different ways of approaching such issues. The first used an experimental design and sought to explain how attitudes were associated with or causally related to personal or social factors. The second was concerned with interpreting and understanding the way one group of women perceived themselves and were perceived by those around them. The two studies reveal the different approaches that can be taken to issues of 'meaning' and interpretation. Box 1 (opposite) summarises the approach and findings of the first study.

The research results revealed relationships between attitudes to poverty and other identified variables. However, on its completion, I felt that I still did not have an understanding of the *meanings* that poverty and unemployment had for all these people or the reasons *why* they held particular views. It was also impossible to determine from the data how far their stated attitudes and values might be expressed in behaviour. Further, the limited conclusions I was able to draw from this research were difficult to convey to the people who had responded to the questionnaire. The study was of interest only to academics. I was left with a profound sense of unease. I knew that there were flaws in the study and I was also convinced that somehow there had to be different ways of working with people that would provide more satisfying and relevant understandings.

In the second study, described in Box 2 (overleaf), I had opportunities to discover and use such methods. Interpretations of the nature of deinstitutionalisation, and of the ways the lived experience of the women in the locked unit was constructed by those around them, flowed from descriptions of the women's lives, and from my experience as a researcher. In contrast with case study A, I was very conscious that in writing up the research I was the interpreter and that different meanings and conclusions could have been drawn.

2   Diverse meanings

My study of attitudes to poverty was grounded in a view of the world that saw the role of research as testing hypotheses derived from theories in

---

Box 1: Case study A – attitudes to poverty

The questions

- What kinds of attitudes to poverty do people have?

- What underlies people's attitudes to poverty?

- How are these attitudes influenced by people's life experiences, socio-economic status, religious or political affiliations and their values?

These questions arose from work in a large welfare agency where I was responsible for a national education programme designed to increase awareness of poverty and unemployment among church members. They led to the development of hypotheses which specified, on the basis of previous research and my work experience, possible relationships between certain variables.

Searching for answers

To test these hypotheses, I designed a large questionnaire, of more than 80 questions, each of which had multiple answers. This was tested for validity and reliability. It was then completed by more than 1000 people who attended church across five different denominations in a particular city. Sophisticated statistical analyses were used to explore the relationship between variables and to explain the diverse views about poverty held by these groups.

Researcher's role

My role was to design the research, conceptualise the hypotheses and the questionnaire, manage the research process and analyse the data. I did not consider discussing the issues with research participants and I did not see my own values and attitudes as part of the research.

Findings

Some relationships between different sets of variables were found, most notably between structural views of poverty, more advanced educational levels and Labour party political affiliation. More judgemental attitudes were associated with low educational levels and Conservative political affiliations. There was no significant relationship between attitudes and values or church affiliation.

(Source: adapted from Johnson, 1984)

---

order to discover relationships between variables assumed by the researcher to be important (Grbich, 1999; Denzin and Lincoln, 1998; Hamilton, 1998; and Chapter 3 of this book). Case study B sought to explore how people saw themselves and each other and how changes in policy and practice affected their perceptions and relationships. And yet both studies were concerned at some level with the meanings people gave to their experience.

Box 2: Case study B – studying the closure of a large hospital for people with learning difficulties

The questions

- How have the policies of community living affected the lives of people with learning difficulties who live in hospitals?

- What is life like for women living in a locked unit in a hospital?

- How are they seen by staff and by themselves?

- What is the impact of hospital closure on these women and those working with them?

Answering these questions led to a four-year project exploring the impact of the closure of a large hospital for people with learning difficulties on a group of women who lived there in a locked unit. They had been labelled as having 'learning difficulties' and 'challenging behaviours'.

Searching for answers

To answer my research questions I was involved in several different research activities over the 20 months I spent with the women, living and working in the locked unit. These included:

- Hundreds of hours in the locked unit, talking with the women and helping with day-to-day tasks.

- Three interviews with each staff member in the unit and interviews with the women's families and advocates.

- Three interviews with each of the people managing the closure of the hospital.

- Attendance at management meetings during the closure.

- Analysis of the women's files.

- Participation in, and observation of, the meetings held with the women and their families during the closure of the hospital, to establish preferences for their future living arrangements.

- Participation in, and observation of, meetings held by professionals who made the final decisions about where the women would live.

Researcher's role

During the research, my role with the women and the staff at the hospital changed from an outsider to an involved and knowledgeable participant in their lives. For some women I became an advocate, for some families and staff I was a source of information and I provided policy papers to the team closing the hospital to assist them in the process.

Findings

My work provided a rich description of life in the locked unit and increased understandings of the way hospital life shaped the behaviour and experiences of the women living there. It also demonstrated the problematic nature of labels such as 'challenging behaviour' or indeed 'learning difficulties' when applied to individuals. The study revealed how hospital closure was influenced by two different ways of thinking: rights and management. And through a feminist analysis, it gave new insights into how women who have been institutionalised are not only locked out of society but also out of their lives as women.

(Source: adapted from Johnson, 1998)

Qualitative research can appear in different guises. Some studies bear a close relationship to case study A in their characteristics; others are much more concerned with a holistic description and analysis of people and their worlds.

Qualitative researchers, in the words of Denzin and Lincoln (1998, p. 3):

... study things in their natural settings, attempting to make sense of, or interpret, phenomena in terms of the meanings people bring to them.

They go on to point out that qualitative researchers can use a wide range of methods, including:

... the studied use and collection of a variety of empirical materials – case study, personal experience, introspective, life story, interview, observational, historical, interactional and visual texts ... .

[They] deploy a wide range of interconnected methods, hoping always to get a better fix on the subject matter at hand.

(Denzin and Lincoln, 1998, p. 3)

This definition gives a sense of the range of different methods used by those who call themselves qualitative researchers but it does not give a sense of the diversity of goals or ideologies which shape such research (see Box 3 overleaf). Three points where such diversity arises are outlined below (see also Denzin and Lincoln, 1998).

The place of theory

Theory is a problematic concept in qualitative research. It can be a key focus or it can be regarded as secondary to the provision of rich descriptions of life experiences. For some researchers it is important to develop theories from the research data which can then be used to influence policy and professional practice. For example, Kyngas and Hentinen's (1995) study of the meanings attached to compliance with treatment by diabetic adolescents was undertaken to develop a theory that would improve subsequent treatment regimes. A replicable methodology

---

Box 3: Reflection 1

Thinking about the two research studies, carried out 10 years apart, raises some issues about research.

The influence of the wider social and political context in shaping the way research is carried out (see, for example, Flax, 1990; Holloway, 1989). In the 10 years between the two research projects I had been strongly influenced by feminism, crossed disciplinary boundaries more than once, studied psychoanalysis, practised action research and become interested in post-modern social theory.

The uncertain relationship between attitudes and behaviour. In the first study, I assumed that attitudes to poverty expressed on the questionnaire would have some validity and be reflected in behaviour. However, there was no way of checking that this was the case. In the second study, I relied on interpretation of longitudinal observations of people's behaviour in specific contexts. There is, however, no final truth or absolute certainty in the findings of this kind of research.

---

establishing validity and reliability is important in such cases. On the other hand, Diamond's (1992) American study of nursing home care for older people aimed to add to our understanding of life in such places and to explore policy implications. His account is personal in that he held a paid position as a worker throughout his research. The development of a generalisable theory was not a high priority in the study.

The researcher's prior theoretical (and sometimes ideological) position shapes the methodology of qualitative research. So, Lewis's (1996) study of race and gender in social work used post-modern theory as a framework for the research and its interpretation and, consistent with this approach, she used discourse analysis as her methodology.

The position of the researcher

To varying degrees, qualitative researchers include the researcher's values, positions and changing roles explicitly as part of the research data. Feminist researchers, for example, have criticised social science researchers for their failure to recognise the importance of gender (and other researcher characteristics) (Harding, 1987; Fine and Gordon, 1992). Oakley (1990), in a now classic study of women's experiences of doctors, advocates strongly the need for women to do such research.

In my study of hospital closure, I was aware of myself as an important part of the research process:

There are many voices in this study, but inevitably they are all heard through my voice. For this reason, if for no other, it was important that I become 'subject' to my own research. The questions I asked, the observations I made, the knowledge and information I gained from others were constructed and interpreted by me as researcher (Steier, 1991; Shakespeare and Atkinson, 1993). Further, examining my own emotional reactions to situations and exploring some of the unconscious means I used to defend myself against the stress of the women's world enabled me to hypothesise about some of the reactions of others in the situation. This was particularly so in interpreting the reactions of the women during the closure process, for they were often not able to articulate their concerns verbally. An examination of my own reactions acted as a signpost to their possible responses (Sinason, 1992).

(Johnson, 1998, p. 11)

Other theorists (Steier, 1991) and researchers (Borland, 1991; Stacey, 1991; Whyte, 1943) support this view on the basis that the researcher reflecting on their own experience is an important part of the data collection and analysis process.

This rationale for the inclusion of my own experience as part of the research in the study of hospital closure is a far cry from the non-involved position I took in the study of attitudes to poverty. As in that case, researchers may choose not to include themselves at all in the research. Bogdan and Taylor's (1992) study of a neo-natal emergency ward, for example, used observation of the ward and interviews with parents and nursing staff to explore the ways in which babies in the ward were viewed and treated. Throughout the process the researchers deliberately kept both a physical and an emotional distance. (See Box 4.)

Box 4: Reflection 2

Whatever position the researcher takes in the research, it is inevitable that it will in some way influence and inform the research process and its results. Feminists have argued (e.g. Oakley, 1990) that, in the past, research claimed as 'objective' was conducted from a male perspective, ignoring gender issues in both its content and implementation, leading to a bias in relation to and a neglect of women's issues and viewpoints. However, counter-criticisms have been made of this position, not only from those who favour a more distant relationship between researchers and the researched. Some feminists have also argued that relaxing formal procedures in research interviews can lead to a false intimacy between researcher and participants and a later betrayal when the researcher uses data in ways not envisaged by the participants who supplied it (Scott, 1999; Stacey, 1991).

The purposes of qualitative research

Qualitative research is used for diverse purposes. Theory building may be the main purpose of some research (as described above), while other studies may describe the lives of people or institutions within society. For some researchers the focus is on individuals, while for others it is on the behaviour and meanings given to their lives by groups. Some qualitative researchers emphasise the empowerment or emancipation of groups who are otherwise marginalised in society. Qualitative research may also be used to evaluate welfare or health programmes (Greene, 1998) or to influence policy processes (Rist, 1998). (See Box 5.)

Box 5: Reflection 3

Qualitative research is both an exciting and a problematic field to work in. I am conscious that my view of it is strongly influenced by a particular set of values and theories with which other qualitative researchers may not be comfortable. For example, a strong commitment to feminist research theory led me to work as an advocate with the women living in the locked unit, to be self-disclosing about my life, and to use my own reflections as part of the data. To judge the worth of qualitative research does demand that the reader give some thought to the theoretical positions from which it has been developed and the purposes of it.

---

3   Diverse methods

Qualitative researchers use diverse methods, most of which involve some form of discussion or interaction between researcher and participants. Observation, for example, is likely to be in the form of participant observation; interviews are likely to involve open-ended questions and a fairly flexible, interactive approach.

Participant observation

Participant observation has been defined as:

> ... unobtrusive, shared or overtly subjective data collection, which involves a researcher spending time in an environment observing behaviour, action and interaction, so that he/she can understand the meanings constructed in that environment and can make sense of everyday life experiences.

(Grbich, 1999, pp. 123–4)

We are all participant observers in our own lives and in the lives of people around us. Some of us, through life experiences or training, are more vigilant or observant than others. Professional practitioners, for example, may be trained to be careful in observing their own world and that of other people and reflecting on their experience. Participant observation uses skills of observation and reflection over time to report in careful detail others' lives and, sometimes, the researcher's reaction to them.

The degree to which the researcher is actively involved in the research situation as a participant varies, depending on both the context and the researcher's position (Grbich, 1999; Vidich and Lyman, 1998). Atkinson and Hammersley (1998) comment that it is hard to pin down a precise definition of participant observation because of this issue. For example, in case study B, I participated actively in the life of the locked unit over time. However, I observed, without active involvement, management committee meetings of the team closing the hospital, discussed controversial issues with some staff informally, and held formal interviews without self-disclosure with others. The degree of my participation varied with the situation.

The example in Box 6 (overleaf) illustrates some of the characteristics of participant observation. It describes a particular world or scene. The observer not only is aware of what is going on but also records it in detail either as it happens or soon after. Yet this is not detached observation. The researcher, in this instance, intervenes directly in what is happening to point out an error. What this field note description reflects is familiarity and engagement with the people and their world. This slow accumulation of detailed description (and personal reflection) serves a purpose not only in describing a world, a culture or the behaviour and interactions of others but also in leading to a developing understanding of this world and how it works. This field note was but one type of record of participant observation in the unit. Others included detailed descriptions of life in the unit, accounts of particular interactions between people, stories of my own work within the unit and reflections on my observations. Poetry, photographs and pictures were included as additional material in field notes.

Neither the definitions of participant observation nor the field note example can convey the excitement of doing research in this manner or, indeed, of reading it. Some of the best studies using participant observation succeed in drawing readers into unfamiliar worlds or help them to see a familiar world in quite different ways. Such studies not only offer a deepened understanding of these worlds but also challenge the attitudes and values of the reader. For example, Goffman's (1961) classic study of life in a psychiatric hospital not only provided insights about the role of 'total' institutions in general but also challenged prevailing views about people with psychiatric illness and the way they were treated in society and in institutional care. Similarly, Bluebond-Lagner (1978) used observations over time in a children's cancer ward of a hospital to explore the lives of the dying children and their reactions to their predicament and to the treatment they received.

Box 6: Participant observation

I arrived in the room where Jane's preferences (for future living after institutional closure) were being considered half-way through the afternoon (by a panel of professionals). Her first preference was for a house in the grounds at Rochester (a hospital). It was hot and the panel members looked exhausted and frustrated both by the work done, and that which remained.

They had spent the day attempting to juggle the more than forty people who wanted a house in the grounds at Rochester with the twenty-one places available. ... when I looked at the whiteboard with its names and houses I realised that Jane's name was not there. I pointed this out to the panel chairperson. The names were checked and concern was expressed by the panel members at the omission particularly because the allocation to houses was now almost set (Field notes).

(Source: Johnson, 1998, p. 115)

However, a word of warning is needed. Participant observation is also a method that can involve the researcher in very difficult ethical and interpersonal issues. These have been well documented in the literature (see, for example, Estroff, 1981; Burgess, 1984; Edgerton, 1991; Hough, 1996). In the fieldwork for case study B, I formed close relationships with other people in the hospital, many of whom were in conflict. This led to me becoming a repository of politically volatile stories from different people, which could not be shared with others, leading at times to a sense of betrayal.

Further, I found myself caught in a dilemma over how far I should become involved in the lives of the women living in the locked unit. Should I provide information about their lives to the people making decisions about their future living arrangements? Should I advocate for and with them? Should I provide families with information about their relative? I saw what I felt to be injustices done to individual women, witnessed violence (on an almost daily basis) and was helpless to prevent either. I was entrusted with stories by staff members, families and advocates, who wanted to be sure that their views were heard, but finally I had to choose among those stories. I arrived at, not so much a true picture, as *my* picture.

Asking questions and listening to people

In everyday life, much of our understanding of ourselves, other people and the world around us comes, as well as from observation, from sharing ideas, listening to people and asking questions. We use these interactions to interpret the meanings other people give to their worlds, although we may not think of it in these terms. Qualitative researchers have developed a range of methods and accompanying skills that explore meanings through asking questions and discussion. The particular method chosen will depend on the context of the research, the characteristics of the participants and the particular position of the researcher. Box 7 suggests how methods may be varied with different groups of people and in different situations.

Box 7: Asking questions and listening to people

Informal discussions

I could not carry out formal interviews with the women who lived in the locked unit. Many of them found it difficult (some impossible) to use spoken language or to concentrate. So I used informal discussions.

Semi-structured interviews

I was interested in innovative programmes developed by staff in the unit and used a carefully designed set of questions to find out from staff how they saw their work and the effect of the programmes. It was important in this instance to be able to compare answers across the group.

Unstructured interviews

I spent many hours talking with parents. While I had identified themes for discussion, the interviews were wide-ranging and individualised since I was interested in the unique experience of each family.

Group interviews

After the consultation process, which would decide where the women went to live once the hospital closed, I interviewed the closure team as a group in a brainstorming session to obtain their views about the positive and negative aspects of the consultation. Group discussion led to new ideas and to opportunities to raise controversial issues. I used individual interviews with the same staff later to identify issues they may have been unwilling to express in a group situation.

Difficulties in interpreting what we observe and what we hear

Regardless of how we observe or ask questions, difficulties arise from both the kinds of information we gain and the ways in which we interpret it. Information will often be ambiguous, fragmented and partial. Informants may not want to reveal things about themselves or their lives. They may also show only aspects of themselves that they see as relevant or pleasing. Sometimes situations or questions may be misunderstood.

Further, the wider political and social context in which we find ourselves will influence how others behave. Such contexts may position the participants in particular ways and determine both what they are willing or able to do or say and how they say it or do it. For example, feminist writers have argued that women's views and issues have often been hidden by using male interviewers and patriarchal research methods. Such factors may influence strongly not only what participants do or say but also what researchers see or hear. For example, in my observations and interviews in the locked unit of the hospital, I was not only a university-based researcher. I was also a parent and a woman: two factors that may well have influenced what others said and did but also what I myself saw and heard.

Qualitative researchers respond to the shifting, ambiguous, fragmented nature of data in several different ways, depending on the values of the researcher and the nature of the research as follows.

- *The researcher may seek to standardise procedures to reduce variability.* In observations, the setting and what is observed are predetermined. In interviews, the role of the interviewer is tightly scripted in an effort to standardise their influence. And the answers or observations are analysed to extract common and often predetermined themes – see, for example, Kai's (1996) study of parents' difficulties and information needs in coping with acute illness in their pre-school children.

- *The researcher may see the richness of interaction and communication itself as the focus for the research.* Here the researcher's role may become part of the study itself. Or the researcher may 'support' the participant to tell their story as an oral history. This work assumes 'that people live storied lives and that telling and retelling one's story helps one understand and create a sense of self' (Marshall and Rossman, 1999, p. 120), particularly where such stories may have been hidden from view: for example, the stories of women (Anderson and Jack, 1991) or people with disabilities (Morris, 1996; Bornat *et al.*, 1999).

- *The researcher may look at how meanings are created as the focus of the research.* Here the focus is not on what the participant in the research is saying so much as on how the people involved construct meanings between them. Scott (1999), for example, uses this focus in an account of working with Caribbean people on health issues, as does Lewis (1996) in her study of how black women social workers constitute their race, gender and class experience in their work.

Constructing and exploring texts

Another method used by qualitative researchers involves the construction or exploration of written texts. Sometimes this is in the form of transcripts from interviews so that 'asking questions and listening to people' blurs into an exploration of how speech is translated into written language. Other forms of texts that may be analysed or constructed by researchers include: policy documents, archival material, journals kept by researchers, field notes, library materials, diaries, photographs, films and videos (Grbich, 1999; Marshall and Rossman, 1999; Hodder, 1998) (see Box 8).

Box 8: Constructing and exploring texts

Reading the women's files, some of which went back more than 50 years, provided a great deal of information about the women: for example, formal assessments, medical reports and reports of violence or aggressive behaviour. But sometimes I learned more about how they were perceived by those around them from the omissions and silences. A note indicating that a woman's father had died was not accompanied by any statements about her possible grief or how her reaction was perceived by staff. A record of one woman breaking 20 windows and then being sent to the locked unit was not placed in a context nor was there any attempt to give reasons for her behaviour. Sometimes the picture of a woman changed according to who made the record. Positive comments about one woman suddenly changed to negative ones. Only after some time did I realise that the handwriting in the file had changed too, indicating that a new member of staff was responsible for her care. The files provided fragments of information about the women's lives over time in the hospital and also recorded the changing and sometimes unchanging nature of care.

Researchers use texts for different purposes. They may want to examine the lives of people in the past and to explore how attitudes towards them may have changed. For example, Bogdan (1988), in a controversial book, used historical textual evidence from books, films, newspapers, advertising and photographs to describe the lives of people with disabilities who performed in circuses and 'freak shows' throughout the nineteenth century. Similarly, Foucault (1980) examined how discourses about psychiatric illness, medical practices and punishment have shifted and changed across time.

Other researchers prefer to focus on what people say or write about their own lives. For example, Biklen (1995), in exploring the gendered experience of teaching, used archival material from the nineteenth century, autobiographies and fiction, as well as interviews and observation to develop her study. Written sources of any kind may simply supplement other methods. To increase my understanding of how the women came into the locked unit, for example, I studied letters (sometimes 20 years old) from parents recording their experiences with their daughters. These yellowing documents recorded both formal assessments of each woman and individual staff impressions and they were important in tracing aspects of each woman's story.

While some qualitative research focuses primarily on just one method, much of it combines methods and engages the researcher in observation, interviews, document analysis and self-reflection. (See Box 9 overleaf.)

Box 9: Reflection 4

There is a certain artificial neatness in suggesting that a researcher decides which method to use and then goes ahead with the research. In fact, methods often change as the researcher's knowledge and questions evolve. This demands a high degree of skill from the researcher to use multiple methods and be flexible enough to move between them. For some researchers the range of methods used is determined by their ideological commitment to particular forms of research, while others are more eclectic in their approach.

---

4   Diverse analyses

Qualitative research tends, by its very nature, to produce volumes of relatively unstructured data which the researcher must decide how to interpret. This, of course, depends on both the nature of the study and the position the researcher (and sometimes the participant) takes to it. In some qualitative research the process of analysis may be explicit early in the research process through the identification of themes or the use of structured methods which shape the analysis. In other research, interpretations may emerge from the immersion of the researcher in fieldwork (Marshall and Rossman, 1999; Crabtree and Miller, 1992).

> Data analysis is the process of bringing order, structure and interpretation to the mass of collected data. It is a messy, ambiguous, time-consuming, creative and fascinating process. It does not proceed in a linear fashion; it is not neat.
>
> Qualitative data analysis is a search for general statements about relationships among categories of data; it builds grounded theory (Strauss and Corbin, 1998). It is the search among data to identify content for ethnographies and for participants' truths.
>
> (Marshall and Rossman, 1999, p. 151)

Not all qualitative researchers would agree with this account of data analysis as it applies to their research but it is a guide to considering how they go about the work of making sense of their data.

Building grounded theory and the constant comparative method

Grounded theory research demonstrates the way in which research analysis and purpose are integrally related. It aims to generate theory grounded in the data and provides researchers with a systematic approach to data analysis. The approach developed from the concerns voiced by Glaser and Strauss (1967) that qualitative research had failed to generate its own theory. They proposed an analytic method, called the *constant comparative method*, which involves the early identification and coding of categories emerging from interviews or fieldwork.

For example, in their classic study of the medical treatment of dying patients, Glaser and Strauss (1967) found that 'social loss' (or the social value of the patient) was a constantly emerging theme in interviews with nurses. They then compared responses from their interviews, to check for similarity with or difference from previous responses. Gradually the category of 'social loss' became more refined as the researchers discovered its characteristics: for example, the importance of patients' age, educational level or occupational status in determining the nurses' perceptions.

The process of comparison and allocation stops when *theoretical saturation* is reached, that is, when each new incident coded can be fitted unproblematically into the existing categories. As the analysis continues, the theoretical properties of a category are developed. This process leads to the development of a theory grounded in systematic research observation, which may be expressed in context-independent language and may then be applicable in other settings. Kyngas and Hentinen's (1995) grounded theory of compliance with medical care by young diabetic people may, for example, also be applied and tested with other forms of medical compliance by similar adolescent or other specified groups of patients.

Practitioners have disagreed about the best way to use grounded theory approaches (Glaser, 1992; Strauss and Corbin, 1990; Strauss, 1987). However, it has become a very attractive research methodology, particularly for those working in health and social welfare (Strauss and Corbin, 1998) because, while using qualitative methods, it is also systematic and capable of later verification by other researchers.

Other ways of making sense of data

Some qualitative research aims to be descriptive rather than generate theory and some, while concerned with theory, may not involve the rigorous systematisation of data involved in grounded theory research. For such research, the identification of themes through an analysis of interviews or field notes may be sufficient and may come late in the process of the research. Sometimes this will involve a subjective judgement by the researcher and sometimes themes may be coded using computer-based data analyses. (For a useful overview of computer-based programs for qualitative data analysis, see Richards and Richards, 1998.)

Material collected for life histories and stories of an individual's life may require difficult methodological and ethical decisions in the process of analysis (Chanfrault-Duchet, 1991; Etter-Lewis, 1991). These include questions of ownership of the story, decisions about the inclusion of sensitive or painful material and issues of confidentiality. Some researchers using this approach take the stories back to the people who originally told them for verification and discussion. This may result in important new learning about meanings and interpretation (Borland, 1991).

Research that focuses on language uses different approaches to exploring meanings. For example, a discourse analyst views 'the language within which experience is framed as not simply describing the world but as, in some sense, constructing it' (Wilkinson and Kitzinger, 1995, p. 3). Researchers using this kind of framework will work with data from small groups or from an individual in a highly intense way. For some researchers the analysis may be primarily linguistic; for others it may be more concerned with the process of interaction between researcher and participant and the shared meanings constructed from this. (See Box 10.)

Box 10: Reflection 5

Some data analysis (such as the study of attitudes to poverty in Box 1) is preset by the design of the research. However, data analysis in other research may be more heuristic, or exploratory, in style. For example, in the hospital closure study (Box 2), several different forms of analysis were used. Decisions about analysis arose from experience. This does not mean I did not consider and use systematic ways of analysing data. I did but it was a heuristic process rather than one that was settled by a fixed view of either research design or data analysis. Sometimes I used key themes from interviews and document analysis; other times I focused strongly on the use of language and on discourses about the women to understand their lives; and sometimes I tried to find ways to give their voices a chance to speak independently.

---

5   Diverse assessments and diverse uses

Because of the diverse meanings of qualitative research and the diversity of its method, assessing and using it requires flexibility and varied means of evaluation by the reader. There are two key questions for health and social welfare practitioners approaching qualitative research:

1 Is this research meaningful, helpful or relevant to me?

2 How far can I trust or rely on this research?

It is probably clear from earlier in this chapter that it is difficult to provide clear answers to these questions. So much depends on the kind of research that is being discussed and the position of the reader. But there are some useful guidelines for assessing and using qualitative research.

Is this research meaningful, helpful or relevant to me?

Judgements tend to be based on the extent to which the research:

- conveys a sense of integrity in relation to the worlds the researcher has explored
- resonates with the reader's own experiences, whether personal or professional, leading either to confirmation or to an acknowledged challenge of such experiences
- leads to the clarification or resolution of problems confronting the individual reader.

For practitioners specifically, other factors may include the extent to which the research:

- provides a basis for self-reflection by practitioners
- provides a theoretical understanding of the ways in which individuals and groups construct or interpret meanings in their lives
- heightens awareness of the ways in which individuals see their own lives and their inclusion in or exclusion from their communities
- changes ways of viewing the world, challenging us not to accept our assumptions or practices as being somehow fixed, coherent and consistent but rather to see much of our social world as shifting, fragmented and subject to change.

How far can I trust or rely on this research?

Evaluating experimental research uses the key criteria of *validity* (does it measure what it says it measures) and *reliability* (can this process be repeated in the same conditions and produce the same result).

While these criteria can still be used for some forms of qualitative research (for example, some grounded theory studies are suited to this kind of evaluation), it is not appropriate for other forms of qualitative research for several reasons.

Some qualitative researchers actually seek to explore the uniqueness of the particular issues they are studying, while others are concerned with documenting the way in which meanings shift, change and are fragmented. It would be paradoxical in this situation to apply criteria that assume continuation and fixedness of meanings. Still other qualitative research seeks to provide the means for people who may otherwise be silenced to have a voice. In these instances, reliability and validity are particularly problematic. For example, how does one assess the validity and reliability of my account of life in a locked unit? How does one assess the 'truth' of a woman's account of her life?

Some writers have sought to find answers to how such research can be assessed. For example, Vidich and Lyman (1998, p. 44) comment:

... we judge for ourselves on the standard of whether the work communicates or 'says' something to us – that is – does it connect with our reality?

Does it provide us with insights that help us organise our own observations? Does it resonate with our image of the world? Or does it provide such a powerful incursion on the latter that we feel compelled to re-examine what we have long supposed to be true about our life world?

This kind of assessment suggests the need to evaluate some forms of qualitative research with criteria that reflect the shifting nature of our realities and are more related to 'trustworthiness' and 'authenticity' (Denzin and Lincoln, 1998, p. 187). Such a view of evaluation of research places responsibility for judging and assessing the worth of a piece of research on the reader and acknowledges that there may be diverse views about the research itself. (See Box 11.)

Box 11: Reflection 6

The study of hospital closure (Box 2) is an example of the different ways of assessing qualitative research.

- It provided detailed descriptions of life in a locked unit and documented the women's lives in an effort to bring this particular world to life.

- It involved interviews with staff, parents and the people closing the hospital as well as documentary analysis. Gaining information from different groups led to some confirmation of ideas (in a process similar to triangulation), revealed differences in meanings and perceptions and led to new theories and ideas, which emerged from a consideration of the total information.

- The voices of the women living in the locked unit and those working closely with them were heard directly in the final document.

Conclusion

Much qualitative research involves an exploration of meanings. It seeks to explore and shed light on the rich, changing and complex worlds of meanings that we construct and interpret through our lives and our experiences with each other. It does not seek to find fixed categories and laws to explain human behaviour but rather to challenge such categories, to question commonly accepted assumptions on which we operate and to explore the diverse ways in which we live together.

To engage with interpreting meanings requires researchers to adopt an explicitly reflective role, recognising their own biases, interests and expectations as well as potential influences on the behaviour and expectations of others. Such awareness and the skills involved in what might be seen as more participative approaches to research have much in common with the skills of critical and reflective practice. Both are concerned with developing better understandings that are trustworthy and relevant and both can feed into and learn from each other.

References

Anderson, K. and Jack, D. C. (1991) 'Learning to listen: interview techniques and analyses', in Gluck, S. B. and Patai, D. (eds) *Women's Words: The Feminist Practice of Oral History*, pp. 11–26, London, Routledge.

Atkinson, P. and Hammersley, M. (1998) 'Ethnography and participant observation', in Denzin, N. K. and Lincoln, Y. S. (eds) *Strategies of Qualitative Inquiry*, pp. 110–36, London, Sage.

Biklen, S. K. (1995) *School Work: Gender and the Cultural Construction of Teaching*, New York, Teachers College Press.

Bluebond-Lagner, M. (1978) *The Private Worlds of Dying Children*, Princeton, NJ, Princeton University Press.

Bogdan, R. (1988) *Freak Show*, Chicago, Chicago University Press.

Bogdan, R. and Taylor, S. (1975) *Introduction to Qualitative Research Methods: A Phenomenological Approach to the Social Sciences*, New York, John Wiley.

Bogdan, R. and Taylor, S. J. (1992) 'Be honest not cruel: staff/parent communication on a neo-natal unit', in Ferguson, P. M., Ferguson, D. L. and Taylor, S. J. (eds) *Interpreting Disability: A Qualitative Reader*, New York, Teacher's College Press, Columbia University.

Borland, K. (1991) ' "That's not what I said", Interpretative conflict in oral history narrative research', in Gluck, S. B. and Patai, D. (eds) *Women's Words: The Feminist Practice of Oral History*, pp. 63–72, London, Routledge.

Bornat, J., Perks, R., Thompson, P. and Walmsley, J. (1999) (eds) *Oral History, Health and Welfare*, London, Routledge.

Burgess, R. G. (1984) *In the Field: An Introduction to Field Research*, London, George Allen and Unwin.

Chanfrault-Duchet, M.-F. (1991) 'Narrative structures, social models and symbolic representation in the life story', in Gluck, S. B. and Patai, D. (eds) *Women's Words: The Feminist Practice of Oral History*, pp. 77–92, London, Routledge.

Crabtree, B. F. and Miller, W. L. (eds) (1992) *Doing Qualitative Research: Multiple Strategies*, Newbury Park, CA, Sage.

Denzin, N. K. and Lincoln, Y. S. (1998) 'Introduction: entering the field of qualitative research', in Denzin, N. K. and Lincoln, Y. S. (eds) *The Landscape of Qualitative Research: Theories and Issues*, pp. 1–34, London, Sage.

Diamond, T. (1992) *Making Gray Gold: Narratives of Nursing Home Care*, Chicago, Chicago University Press.

Edgerton, R. B. (1991) *Lives of Older People with Mental Retardation in the Community*, Maryland, Paul H. Brookes.

Estroff, S. (1981) *Making it Crazy: An Ethnography of Psychiatric Patients in an American Community*, Berkeley, CA, University of California Press.

Etter-Lewis, G. (1991) 'Black women's life stories: reclaiming self in narrative texts', in Gluck, S. B. and Patai, D. (eds) *Women's Words: The Feminist Practice of Oral History*, pp. 43–58, London, Routledge.

Fine, M. and Gordon, S. M. (1992) 'Feminist transformations of/despite psychology', in Fine, M. (ed.) *Disruptive Voices: The Possibilities of Feminist Research*, Ann Arbor, University of Michigan Press.

Flax, J. (1990) *Thinking Fragments: Psychoanalysis, Feminism and Postmodernism in the Contemporary West*, Berkeley, University of California Press.

Foucault, M. (1980) *Power/Knowledge: Selected Interviews and Other Writings 1972–1977*, New York, Harvester Wheatsheaf.

Glaser, B. (1992) *Basics of Grounded Theory Analysis*, California, Sociology Press.

Glaser, B. and Strauss, A. (1967) *The Discovery of Grounded Theory*, Chicago, Aldine.

Goffman, E. (1961) *Asylums: Essays on the Social Situation of Mental Patients and Other Inmates*, London, Peregrine Books.

Grbich, C. (1999) *Qualitative Research in Health*, London, Sage.

Greene, J. (1998) 'Qualitative program evaluation', in Denzin, N. K. and Lincoln, Y. S. (eds) *Collecting and Interpreting Qualitative Materials*, pp. 372–99, London, Sage.

Hamilton, D. (1998) 'Traditions, preferences and postures in applied qualitative research', in Denzin, N. K. and Lincoln, Y. S. (eds) *The Landscape of Qualitative Research: Theories and Issues*, pp. 111–29, London, Sage.

Harding, S. (1987) 'Is there a feminist method?', in Harding, S. (ed.) *Feminism and Methodology: Social Science Issues*, Milton Keynes, Open University Press.

Hodder, I. (1998) 'The interpretation of documents and material culture', in Denzin, N. K. and Lincoln, Y. S. (eds) *Collecting and Interpreting Qualitative Materials*, pp. 110–29, London, Sage.

Holloway, W. (1989) *Subjectivity and Method in Psychology*, London, Sage.

Hough, G. (1996) 'Using ethnographic methods to research the work world of social workers in child protection', in Fook, J. (ed.) *The Reflective Researcher: Social Workers' Theories of Practice Research*, pp. 43–54, St Leonards, Allen and Unwin.

Johnson, K. (1984) 'Attitudes to poverty among Christian groups', unpublished MA thesis, University of Melbourne.

Johnson, K. (1998) *Deinstitutionalising Women: An Ethnographic Study of Institutional Closure*, Cambridge, Cambridge University Press.

Kai, J. (1996) 'Parents' difficulties and information needs in coping with acute illness in pre-school children: a qualitative study', *British Medical Journal*, Vol. 313, pp. 987–90.

Kyngas, H. and Hentinen, M. (1995) 'Meaning attached to compliance with self-care, and conditions for compliance among young diabetics', *Journal of Advanced Nursing*, Vol. 21, pp. 729–36.

Lewis, G. (1996) 'Situated voices: "Black women's experience" and social work', *Feminist Review*, Vol. 53, pp. 24–56.

Marshall, C. and Rossman, G. B. (1999) *Designing Qualitative Research* (3rd edn), London, Sage.

Morris, J. (ed.) (1996) *Encounters with Strangers: Feminism and Disability*, London, The Women's Press.

Oakley, A. (1990) 'Interviewing women: a contradiction in terms', in Roberts, H. (ed.) *Doing Feminist Research*, pp. 30–61, London, Routledge.

Richards, T. and Richards, L. (1998) 'Using computers in qualitative research', in Denzin, N. K. and Lincoln, Y. S. (eds) *Collecting and Interpreting Qualitative Materials*, pp. 211–45, London, Sage.

Rist, R. (1998) 'Influencing the policy process with qualitative research', in Denzin, N. K. and Lincoln, Y. S. (eds) *Collecting and Interpreting Qualitative Materials*, pp. 400–23, London, Sage.

Scott, P. (1999) 'Black people's health: ethnic status and research issues', in Hood, S., Mayall, B. and Oliver, S. (eds) *Critical Issues in Social Research Power and Prejudice*, pp. 80–93, Buckingham, Open University Press.

Shakespeare, P. and Atkinson, D. (1993) 'Introduction', in Shakespeare, P., Atkinson, D. and French, S. (eds) *Reflecting on Research Practice: Issues in Health and Social Welfare*, pp. 1–10, Buckingham, Open University Press.

Sinason, V. (1992) *Mental Handicap and the Human Condition*, New Approaches from the Tavistock Series, London, Free Association Books.

Stacey, J. (1991) 'Can there be a feminist ethnography?', in Gluck, S. B. and Patai, D. (eds) *Women's Words: The Feminist Practice of Oral History*, pp. 111–20, London, Routledge.

Steier, F. (1991) 'Introduction: research as self-reflexivity, self-reflexivity as social process', in Steier, F. (ed.) *Research and Reflexivity*, pp. 1–11, London, Sage.

Strauss, A. L. (1987) *Qualitative Analysis for Social Scientists*, Cambridge, Cambridge University Press.

Strauss, A. and Corbin, J. (1990) *Basics of Qualitative Research*, California, Sage.

Strauss, A. and Corbin, J. (1998) 'Grounded theory methodology: an overview', in Denzin, N. K. and Lincoln, Y. S. (eds) *Strategies of Qualitative Inquiry*, pp. 158–83, London, Sage.

Vidich, A. J. and Lyman, S. M. (1998) 'Qualitative methods: their history in sociology and anthropology', in Denzin, N. K. and Lincoln, Y. S. (eds) *The Landscape of Qualitative Research*, pp. 41–109, London, Sage.

Whyte, W. F. (1943) *Street Corner Society: The Social Structure of an Italian Slum*, Chicago, University of Chicago Press.

Wilkinson, S. and Kitzinger, C. (1995) (eds) *Feminism and Discourse: Psychological Perspectives*, London, Sage.

Chapter 5
Using action research

Elizabeth Hart and Meg Bond

Introduction

Some research is designed to generate knowledge without at the time directly altering the phenomena being studied. Much survey research falls into this category. So, too, do some qualitative research projects. Other research, however, starts with a commitment to change and the logic of its design and its strategies and procedures are very much premised on the notion of working towards change. Action research, as the term implies, falls into this category. The aim of this chapter is to explore some of the major forms of action research, document ways in which they have been used in the health and social care field, and assess the arguments of its supporters and detractors.

1   Defining action research

Action research aims to contribute to the practical concerns of people in an immediate problematic situation and to the goals of social science by joint collaboration within a mutually acceptable ethical framework.
(Rapoport, 1970, p. 499)

Action research is undertaken by participants in social situations to improve their practices and their understanding of them.
(Bowling, 1997, p. 366)

These two definitions, written over a quarter of a century apart, demonstrate strong continuities in thinking about the aims of action research. Both definitions see it as essentially practical – enabling practitioners to deal with problems of immediate concern in their everyday work situations. Also, both definitions are underpinned by the assumption that change and improvement are on the agenda, and that the aim is not simply to produce 'academic' theory. But they also highlight areas of difference. Rapoport's classic definition assumes that two parties are involved in solving the problem – managers on the one hand, and social scientists on the other. The situation thus requires collaboration between the very different cultures of the managerial and academic worlds and 'gives rise to issues about whether the aims of the work will be concerned primarily with problem-solving for the particular organization, or with producing theoretical generalizations ... ' (Gill and Johnson, 1991, p. 60).

In Bowling's definition, by contrast, the focus is much more on practitioners – whether they be health service managers, nurses, therapists or social care workers – engaging in action research for the purpose of improving their knowledge base and their practice. In this case, there is no separation between practitioner and academic researcher; the emphasis is on all those with a stake in resolving the problem being participants in the change process. Moreover, the contributions to knowledge that are envisaged are concerned with practitioners' improved understandings of the problems of their practice, and not with the development of social science theory.

This latter emphasis is illustrated in the following definition, which extends to include problem solving in organisations and communities.

> Action research is research that provides practitioners, organizations or communities with the tools to solve their problems. ... Action research is rooted in practice, organizational or community issues as articulated by non-academic researchers, and addresses issues that a community, practitioner or organization actually experiences and wants to resolve. The research process is marked by collaboration with community organizations and groups in a cyclical investigation of agreed upon problems.
>
> (Boutilier *et al.*, 1997, p. 70)

The seven criteria outlined in Box 1 (overleaf) were developed as a way of distinguishing action research from other approaches. When applying these criteria to specific instances, however, as we do in Section 3, it is important to remember that it is not any single criterion on its own but the dynamic interplay between them that gives action research its distinctive character. All research methodologies, for example, are educative in a broad sense because they aim to increase knowledge. A clinical trial involves an intervention which may change practice, and it would be difficult to find a researcher who did research to make things worse! The distinctiveness of action research lies in its concern to enable learning to take place as part of a process of change and improvement, and in dealing with problems in the social contexts of people's lives.

2   Origins and development

Kurt Lewin (1890–1947) is widely recognised for introducing the term 'action research'. Lewin was a psychologist of Prussian origin, who emigrated to America in the early 1930s to escape the Nazi persecution of Jewish people. As a student in Berlin, Lewin had been active in left-wing politics, and was committed to improving the lives of working class people by making the factory system much more humane and democratic. Even a

---

Box 1: Features of action research

1   Is educative.

2   Deals with individuals as members of social groups.

3   Focuses on problems in their social context.

4   Is informed by a cyclical framework.

5   Involves a change intervention in which there is a complex interplay between research and action.

6   Is concerned with involvement and improvement.

7   Is collaborative and involves participants in the process as change agents.

(Source: adapted from Hart and Bond, 1995a, pp. 37–8)

---

quick glance through the action research literature shows how important Lewin's influence has been. Yet he wrote relatively little about action research. He developed the approach late in his career, in about 1944, and died before he could see the outcome of his planned action research experiments in industrial participation (Adelman, 1993).

Lewin's main concern was to understand the impact of membership of a social group on individuals' views and attitudes. He believed that social facts were no less real than physical facts, and could be studied objectively by experimental means. He believed that social groups could be harnessed to change behaviour in a way that was not possible by appeal to the individual alone. In a chapter entitled 'Action research and minority problems' (Lewin, 1948), he describes action research as a way of marrying the experimental method with social action and responding to major social problems of the day (Kemmis *et al.*, 1982). Using what he termed the 'change experiment', Lewin pioneered the transfer of the experimental method of the natural sciences to the social sciences (Allport, 1948). Others have elaborated his approach in different ways (Box 2 opposite).

Figure 1 (overleaf) illustrates the nature of action research. It shows a cyclical process, representing Lewin's concept of action research as a 'spiral of steps' (Lewin, 1948, p. 207). This idea has formed the basis of many later definitions of action research (Meyer, 1993), although different writers use somewhat different terms.

The process begins with diagnosing (at the top) – for example, identifying the problem. As discussed in Section 5, this is not as simple as it sounds, and here Lewin's approach can be particularly helpful. In Lewin's terms, problem identification involves exploring what he termed a *general idea*, which may simply mean a 'gut feeling' that a particular area of practice could be improved in some way. This is followed by *fact finding*, which might involve analysing case notes or checking out with colleagues, talking to clients and reading around the area. Fact finding clarifies the

---

Box 2: Some key contributors to action research

Jaques (1951) – is representative of the Tavistock Institute school of organisational action research which focuses on workplace group dynamics. It involves a commitment to establishing relationships with clients over time, an emphasis on research as a social process, a concern with implementation and change, as well as the generation of social science theory. Psychoanalytic theory contributes to ideas about working with and through conflict.

Susman and Evered (1978) – argue that positivist science fails to respond to the challenges of problem solving in complex human organisations. Action researchers can act as catalysts working with people to define and resolve problems. Issues of process are considered as important as issues of outcomes.

Carr and Kemmis (1986) – suggest that contemporary action researchers regard group decision-making as essential for authentic commitment to social action. Action research is seen as an embodiment of democratic principles of research, promoting critiques of oppressive social conditions. Action research is concerned with improving rather than proving.

Adelman (1993) – considers that improvements in practice depend on bringing together the strands of organisational change, democratic practice, group process and reflective practice in a methodological framework of participatory research.

Shuttleworth *et al.* (1994) – assess the extent and nature of 'collaborative' research, particularly studies bringing together workers and academics in shared research projects. They argue that imbalances in power relations contribute to a major contradiction between the outsider professional researcher's role in introducing ideas and planning a shared learning process, and the insider participants' abilities to influence the development and framing of emergent knowledge.

---

general idea and may even involve a complete rethink – meaning more fact finding and analysis.

Moving around the cycle clockwise highlights the need for *action planning*, and for selecting an intervention. This process is well illustrated in case study 2 in Section 3, which shows how a multidisciplinary team went about the task of selecting patient-centred goal planning as the focus of their overall improvement strategy. For any problem, there may be several possible approaches: thus, when selecting interventions, account needs to be taken of such things as the time available, the scale of the problem, the learning needs of participants and the level of funding provided.

The next step, *action taking*, is about implementing the selected intervention to bring about change – for example, piloting patient-centred goal planning. Moving on, *evaluating* is integral to the change

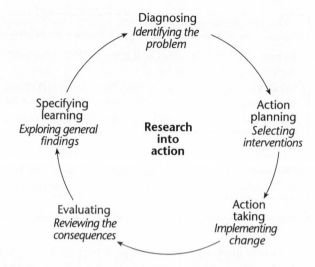

Figure 1   **Cycle of action research** (Source: adapted from Susman and Evered, 1978, in East and Robinson, 1994, p. 58)

process in action research and, when selecting an intervention, it is important to consider how it might be evaluated. However, as Figure 1 shows, the process does not stop at evaluating because this can lead to *specifying learning*, which then propels the change process into a new cycle of *diagnosing*, and so on.

One of the strengths of an action research framework of this kind is that it enables enthusiasm for change to be channelled and sustained beyond the initial idea. This is particularly clear in case study 2 later, where previous attempts by the team to implement change had floundered because they relied on enthusiasm alone to carry them forward. Another strength of the framework is that it allows time for taking stock, reviewing and reflecting, which can be very helpful when projects reach the 'don't know what to do next' phase. Garside (1998, p. s14) argues that many organisations fail at the implementation stage:

> Lack of momentum for the change process or project as it enters the middle phase of its projected lifespan is a common cause of failure to implement. Projects begin with much enthusiasm, momentum, and elaborate project management flow charts but if momentum is not maintained through the critical phase half or two thirds of the way through the process, then even with political and top support in place, the process can flounder.

Most types of change do not happen overnight, and final outcomes cannot be mapped out clearly beforehand (Collins, 1998). For Lewin this was why evaluation of each action step was so important, because otherwise it would not be possible either to alter course in response to changing circumstances or to modify the objective in the light of consequences of an action step. He points out:

If we cannot judge whether an action has led forward or backward, if we have no criteria for evaluating the relation between effort and achievement, there is nothing to prevent us from making the wrong conclusions.

(Lewin, 1948, p. 202)

Lewin argues there is little point in holding a community meeting about how to deal with racial discrimination in the local area, for example, if the only evidence on which to evaluate its achievement was the feelings of the community workers. He likened such an approach to the captain of a ship who, on realising that the ship has veered too far in the wrong direction, turns the steering wheel sharply in the opposite direction, and then goes off to dinner, leaving the ship to go round in circles.

In the next section, four case studies of action research are described and briefly discussed. Each of them is underpinned by the framework discussed above, and yet each of them is very different in character.

3   Four examples of action research

Case study 1 (Box 3 overleaf) is a particularly clear example of a study that fits Rapoport's definition of action research in Section 1. On the one hand, there are the goals of the people with the problem and, on the other, there are the goals of the researcher. The first set of goals is concerned with practical problem solving and the second with the development of social science theory. As is characteristic of this *organisational action research*, the roles of researchers and practitioners were clearly differentiated. The researchers were a university-based expert on theoretical knowledge and its application and a consultant and co-ordinator for the development project, and staff worked 'under the guidance and supervision of researchers' (Lauri and Sainio, 1998, p. 425). Nevertheless, there was certainly an element of collaboration in the sense outlined in the final criterion of Box 1. Physicians and nurse managers were part of the project team, and the nursing staff implementing the care programme were treated as participants in the change process, their views being considered alongside the patients' views.

Because the aim of the project was to improve the care of breast cancer patients rather than to test a specific treatment, it was primarily concerned with organisational change. The intervention involved several levels: the way in which nurses interacted with staff (behavioural change); the content of the care programme itself (technical change); and how patient care was organised (systemic change). In order to carry through organisational change of this kind, the co-operation and commitment of the project team is essential, as too is that of the practitioners whose practice is under review, although the separation of the roles of practitioner and researcher can give rise to problems. This might explain why the evaluation of the nurses' views of the programme highlighted

Box 3: Case study 1 – developing the nursing care of breast cancer patients

This study was designed to use action research to improve the nursing care of breast cancer patients at a hospital in Finland. A novel intervention was established and implemented on the oncology units and surgical wards over a period of 12 months. The programme had three dimensions: (1) information sheets on a range of matters, including the disease and its treatment over time, what the operation involved, post-operative pain, and diet and healthy eating advice; (2) the development of a specific care programme for breast cancer patients; and (3) the strong commitment of relevant staff to improved co-operation between units and wards.

Two surveys at the hospital established a baseline from which to evaluate any improvement resulting from the change. One survey analysed evidence from 100 case notes about breast cancer patients' pathways through the hospital, and the other analysed interview data from 40 new breast cancer patients about their experiences of the hospital system and information needs over time. The findings from these two surveys showed that care was uncoordinated – cancer patients were being moved about between surgery and oncology, and saw several different professionals during their stay. Although patients received more information than those in an earlier study, there was a particular lack of information about the emotional aspects of coping with cancer.

An action research team was established, consisting of nurses, physicians and directors of nursing from both oncology and surgery, plus the two researchers. A theoretical model developed by the researchers was then put together with the empirical data from the two baseline studies to construct a 12-month development programme. Evaluation was done through two questionnaires to measure the information that patients received and how they were coping emotionally. A total of 96 patients were included in this part of the project.

Over half of the patients said they had not received sufficient information before admission to the surgical ward, and about half of the patients in the oncology clinic had received no information at all about important health care issues such as diet and vitamins. Patients also reported problems with privacy and with nursing staff, although the majority recognised that staff had provided information and support to help alleviate their fears of surgery and, of these, almost two-thirds thought this was important. Nursing staff on the two units differed in their views, those on the surgical side feeling more positive about the programme as a learning experience, which they felt improved the care they gave. Half of these believed that the change brought about by the intervention would be permanent. In oncology there were mixed views, some staff claiming that the programme was disorganised and time-consuming, while others felt it helped them generate new ideas about how to organise their work.

(Source: adapted from Lauri and Sainio, 1998)

communication problems, including criticism of how the project was managed by the researchers. It might also explain the differences of view between the oncology and surgery nurses about the positive benefits of the project.

Case study 2 (Box 4) demonstrates a rather different approach to the interplay of research and action and to collaboration, with professionals committing themselves to changing and improving their own practice.

This case study is particularly useful because it exemplifies the use of the action research spiral to think through the steps in a project, and to build in phases of reflection and review. Previously, carried along by their

---

Box 4: Case study 2 – enhancing team functioning in a neuro-rehabilitation team

This project involved a large multidisciplinary team at the Northern General Hospital in Sheffield providing specialist rehabilitation to patients with a brain injury. The team combined nursing, physiotherapy, occupational therapy, communication therapy, art and music therapy, medicine, psychology and social work. They had already spent some time developing specialist expertise and skills and, with the introduction of clinical audit, had given some thought to how they might improve their effectiveness and efficiency. The team wanted to find ways of working together more collaboratively and improving outcomes for patients.

The project used a system of patient-centred goal planning, building on a process developed by a similar team at the Rivermead Rehabilitation Centre in Oxford. After reading published accounts, and obtaining further documentation, five team members attended a workshop run by the Rivermead Centre on the process of goal planning. After a feedback session, the team agreed to adopt this approach. A programme of regular meetings was planned to examine the goal-planning process in more detail and to practise setting aims, objectives and targets. It was agreed that the Life Goals Questionnaire, part of the assessment strategy developed by the Rivermead team, should be completed with all new patients on admission, and that the nursing staff would do this activity. The first case would be reviewed two weeks after admission, and immediately before this the team would discuss information from the Life Goals Questionnaire with the purpose of focusing the review on the patient's goals.

A second delegation of team members attended a further Rivermead workshop with the aim of obtaining information relevant to their needs. Feedback from the second workshop was very encouraging, and subsequent meetings enabled the team to clarify the process of goal planning further. The team decided to use the patient-centred goal plans with 10 consecutive patients, and then to review the outcome.

(Source: adapted from Bennett, 1998)

enthusiasm, the team had tried to introduce changes in an unsystematic way. This time they began by identifying a *general idea*: how to make their weekly multidisciplinary team meetings more focused, disciplined and less wasteful of their time. At this point they were actively engaged in *diagnosing* the problem, which included exploring the possibility of tackling it through patient-centred goal planning, and finding out more about such forms of planning. The team then agreed to incorporate patient-centred goal planning into their practice, and the *first action step* was to attend a workshop to learn about the process.

At this stage, the general idea was not fixed – after the first workshop, the team may have decided this was not the way forward after all. By meeting after the first workshop, the five delegates could evaluate the results of the first action step, before discussion with the rest of the team. At the full meeting (the *second action step*), the team took the opportunity to reflect on earlier failures and to learn from them, and to stimulate discussion, check for consensus and conflict within the team, with the aim of moving things on. As a result the team decided patient-centred goal planning would be central to their strategy. It was then time to plan the next action step and, as part of this, to do some fact finding about how best to evaluate the intervention. The planned programme of team meetings to examine and learn about the goal-planning process in more detail, was the *third action step*.

In terms of the action research cycle (Figure 1), the team had been *action planning*. They began *action taking* when they started implementing the change by piloting the new system. Action planning takes time. The team had to learn new skills and techniques and gain confidence with the process, as well as learn how to work together in a more collaborative way, and this in turn led them to specify further learning needs, which they met by sending another delegation to a second Rivermead workshop.

If case study 1 exemplifies organisational action research and the separation of roles, case study 2, where practitioners are in the lead, can perhaps be thought of as *professionalising* action research. Case study 3 (Box 5 opposite) is an example of both an *empowering* type of action research and practitioner research, to which it is closely allied. It was informed by a feminist approach, which sought the involvement and collaboration of five mothers, most of whom had discovered that their children had been sexually abused, as well as Pat (a child protection social worker), Tess (a local authority group worker), plus Meg, a course tutor on Pat's MA programme. This was a collaborative group, sharing roles as co-researchers and co-change agents.

Problem identification was not owned by one side or the other – researcher or client – but was jointly owned. As Pat explains:

> The starting point for this research was frustration and optimism. The frustration was with the way in which statutory intervention processes designed to protect children seem to add to the distress and damage

---

Box 5: Case study 3 – working with non-abusing mothers in cases of child abuse

Pat, a child protection social worker, wanted to work with colleagues to change the way they tended to deal with 'non-abusing mothers' as if they were somehow to blame for what had happened to their children. Research had shown that attitudes of this kind tended to be counter-productive for children and non-abusing adults alike. As part of her work on a Masters programme, Pat ran a series of focus groups involving five women, four of them mothers of children who had been sexually abused, and Tess, a local authority group worker. The women met each other through a support group started by Tess, and the group became known as the 'For Mothers By Mothers Group'. The women collaborated over a two-year period, and initiatives from the project are still ongoing.

The project provided an opportunity to gain a better understanding of the process of 'blaming' mothers, and to identify barriers to, and opportunities for, working more constructively with them. Focus groups were the chosen method both because of the scope to generate data, and because of the opportunity to stimulate action and to offer women support through the research process itself. Outcomes included a booklet, 'For Mothers By Mothers', to be handed out by social workers at the beginning of statutory investigations, which, after piloting, was to be available for sale. A joint funding bid to pilot a therapeutic and support group for mothers was prepared; links were made with students on other courses who also wanted to improve practice in respect of non-abusing mothers; and plans were made for collective user involvement in an advanced child protection studies programme. Interestingly, the source from which this summary is drawn came from a shared conference presentation, showing how practitioners and users can work together to improve services and develop policy in child protection.

(Source: adapted from Bond *et al.*, 1998)

---

already caused to them by being sexually abused by a loved and trusted adult. ... The optimism was associated with a belief that things could be different ...

(Bond *et al.*, 1998, p. 115)

Four of the mothers (Angela, Bev, Gill and Myrna) add:

Basically, we wanted to be involved in changing what we felt was wrong with the services, and to let the services know what we felt they did right, what helped us most and what was lacking. When we all discovered the abuse of our children, we found there was no information out there, nobody to supply any sort of information apart from academic books, which really in our confused states were not a help.

(Bond *et al.*, 1998, p. 115)

From the very beginning of this project, change and improvement were on the agenda. As is usual in the empowering type of action research, this involved an educative project that enhanced user-control, shifting the balance of power away from social workers and towards users, giving them a voice when before no one had listened to them. The mothers expressed their surprise that the social workers did not seem to know much about people like them and were 'nervous'. 'It was a very strange situation to be in', they said, 'for us to be teaching them' (Bond *et al.*, 1998, p. 119). But they also recognised Pat's key role (p. 116):

> She was like a god-send to us. There was somebody there that could actually put our experiences into words for us and they fitted with the research that we now know about from other countries. That has made people listen and realise that we knew what we were talking about.

Pat herself makes a different comment (p. 121):

> I want to stress the importance for the work of its link with this University programme of social work education. I looked to the institution to help me carry out a rigorous piece of research and to make what I had to say credible. As a result colleagues now listen to what we have to say. Additionally, opportunities continue to be offered to us to present our findings, which is important for raising the awareness of professionals and the public ...

Working in this way – to engage with users, share understandings and learn from and with them – is not an easy option. For practitioners it means letting go of power and status, and being prepared to challenge current practice – both their own and their colleagues' – and in Pat's case she also needed to get her managers on board. However, the change process was immeasurably enhanced by the collaboration, and the ongoing success of the project in propelling other change initiatives is testimony to the strength of this empowering type of action research.

Whereas case study 1 is a fairly large-scale project, carried out by funded professional researchers whose role was clearly separated from that of the practitioners, case studies 2 and 3 are examples of fairly small-scale work linked to practitioner projects. Case study 4 (Box 6 opposite) returns to the larger scale.

This project is a controlled trial (see Chapter 3). However, it may also be seen as an example of Lewin's *experimental type* of action research in that it applies an experimental method to a pressing social problem of the day and involves working with and empowering subjects.

Case study 4 illustrates how the empowering ethos of action research can underpin an experimental design, so that it also becomes possible to measure the impact of a change intervention using standard statistical procedures. In terms of the seven criteria of action research (Box 1), this was an educative project in two senses. First, it required the intervention group of health visitors to learn a new way of working with their clients, one that shifted the balance of power more towards the user. Secondly, it involved families as participants in a learning process about their own problem-solving capabilities and gave them more control over their own lives. It also dealt with families not solely as research subjects, isolated

---

Box 6: Case study 4 – targeting health visiting

Six health authorities were involved in a study aiming to find out whether health visitors who used a structured approach to empower parents to find solutions to their own problems, rather than giving general advice, would positively affect the home environment and developmental levels of infants. The programme focused on more than 1000 families in the UK and Ireland, living in areas of social stress. It involved 86 health visitors, 46 as intervention visitors (who would use the empowering approach) and 40 in the control group (who would advise parents in the usual way). Health visitors from each of the six health authorities were invited to volunteer to take part in the study and, from these, intervention and control health visitors were randomly selected. The children were also selected randomly from each health visitor's own case load. The intervention group of health visitors was trained in the programme methods and enjoined to work with families and encourage them, as far as possible, to find their own solutions to their problems. The control group of health visitors continued with families in the normal way. Each intervention family received monthly visits over a period of two years.

At the beginning, middle and end of the two-year period, a team of specially trained interviewers assessed the home environment and developmental level of each child. The assessment interviews lasted two hours and used a battery of instruments, some specially developed for the programme. This enabled a broad range of areas to be assessed, and included 28 separate items composing a global language score reflecting the child's communication competence. Scores were statistically adjusted to reflect the ages of the children. In total, four million items of evaluation information were gathered, coded and analysed over a four-year period.

The findings showed that the programme had made significant changes in the home environment and developmental level of children from the intervention group, compared with families in the control group. The findings also showed that, for the intervention families, changes in the mothers' self-esteem had been the most significant contributor to the changes in the children. This indicated that enabling the mothers to recognise their own value was essential for progress to be made in influencing children's developmental levels.

(Source: adapted from Barker, 1992)

---

from their everyday social environment, but as members of social groups and communities.

While some might not regard this as an exemplar of action research, its author certainly does. Barker argues that, through designs such as these, action research can take account of what are often thought of as 'soft' data, such as people's own experiences of learning and change. He comments:

What is important here – and this again reflects the action research approach – is the honesty of the relationship between the researchers and the people who are the subjects of the research. In an open relationship, in which people do not feel pressured to report success, it should be possible to gain almost as high a level of both valid and honest reporting as in any double blind trial.

(Barker, 1992, pp. 253–4)

4   Different types of action research

In presenting the case studies as examples of the four different types of action research – organisational, professionalising, empowering and experimental – the notion of different 'types' of action research has emerged. This section explores these different forms of action research further by reference to a typology linking them to the action research criteria in Box 1 (Hart and Bond, 1995a).

The typology locates the four broad types of action research on a continuum in relation to two alternative models of society: a consensus model to the left and a conflict model to the right (Table 1 opposite). It also, harking back to Box 2, suggests that each of the four types has rather different origins. The experimental type has its sources in Lewin's attempt to apply the experimental method of the social sciences to social problems. The organisational type has grown out of an interest in 'bottom-up' approaches to organisational change and problem solving, such as those associated with the Tavistock Institute. The professionalising type is informed by an agenda grounded in practice, reflecting the aspirations of professions such as nursing and social work. The empowering type is most closely associated with community development and is characterised by an explicit anti-oppressive stance to working with vulnerable groups in society. In practice, no project sits neatly in one type, since its focus may shift over time, and it may go through phases where it moves between one type and another.

Focusing on just three of the seven criteria in the typology will indicate its value in drawing attention to key features of the research. Regarding the *educative base*, the typology indicates that within the experimental type the emphasis is on changing people's behaviour through re-education, that is, social engineering. In the organizational type, however, the concern is to overcome resistance to change through education or training; whereas in the professionalising type, the focus is on reflective practice, so that the educative process is grounded in professional knowledge and everyday experience. By the time we get to the empowering type, the educative base has shifted radically and now takes the form of consciousness raising.

Table 1 Action research typology

Action research type: Distinguishing criterion	Consensus model of society Rational social management *Experimental*	*Organisational*	*Professionalising*	Conflict model of society Structural change *Empowering*
1 Educative base	Re-education Enhancing social science/administrative control and social change towards consensus Inferring relationship between behaviour and output; identifying causal factors in group dynamics Social science bias/researcher-focused	Re-education/training Enhancing managerial control and organisational change towards consensus Overcoming resistance to change/restructuring balance of power between managers and workers Managerial bias/client-focused	Reflective practice Enhancing professional control and individual's ability to control work situation Empowering professional groups; advocacy on behalf of patients/clients Practitioner-focused	Consciousness raising Enhancing user-control and shifting balance of power; structural change towards pluralism Empowering oppressed groups User/practitioner-focused
2 Individuals in groups	Closed group, controlled, selection made by researcher for purpose of measurement/inferring relationship between cause and effect Fixed membership	Work groups and/or mixed groups of managers and workers Selected membership	Professional(s) and/or (interdisciplinary) professional group/negotiated team boundaries Shifting membership	Fluid groupings, self-selecting or natural boundary or open/closed by negotiation Fluid membership
3 Problem focus	Problem emerges from the interaction of social science theory and social problems Problem relevant for social science/management interests Success defined in terms of social science	Problem defined by most powerful group; some negotiation with workers Problem relevant for management/social science interests Success defined by sponsors	Problem defined by professional group; some negotiation with users Problem emerges from professional practice/experience Contested, professionally determined definitions of success	Emerging and negotiated definition of problem by less powerful group(s) Problem emerges from members' practice/experience Competing definitions of success accepted and expected

(continued)

Table 1 *(continued)*

	Consensus model of society Rational social management			Conflict model of society Structural change
Action research type:	*Experimental*	*Organisational*	*Professionalising*	*Empowering*
Distinguishing criterion				
4 Change intervention	Social science, experimental intervention to test theory and/or generate theory Problem to be solved in terms of research aims	Top-down, directed change towards predetermined aims Problem to be solved in terms of management aims	Professionally-led, predefined, process-led Problem to be resolved in the interests of research-based practice and professionalisation	Bottom-up, undetermined, process-led Problem to be explored as part of process of change, developing an understanding of meanings of issues in terms of problem and solution
5 Improvement and involvement	Towards controlled outcome and consensual definition of improvement	Towards tangible outcome and consensual definition of improvement	Towards improvement in practice defined by professionals and on behalf of users	Towards negotiated outcomes and pluralist definitions of improvement: account taken of vested interests
6 Cyclic processes	Research components dominant Identifies causal processes that can be generalised Time-limited, task-focused	Action and research components in tension; action-dominated Identifies causal processes that are specific to problem context and/or can be generalised Discrete, rationalist, sequential	Research and action components in tension; research-dominated Identifies causal processes that are specific to problem and/or can be generalised Spiral of cycles, opportunistic, dynamic	Action components dominant Change cause of events; recognition of multiple influences upon change Open-ended, process-driven
7 Research relationship, degree of collaboration	Experimenter/respondents Outside researcher as expert/research funding Differentiated roles	Consultant/researcher, respondent/participants Client pays an outside consultant – 'they who pay the piper call the tune' Differentiated roles	Practitioner or researcher/collaborators Outside resources and/or internally generated Merged roles	Practitioner researcher/co-researchers/co-change agents Outside resources and/or internally generated Shared roles

In terms of *problem focus*, in the experimental type of action research the problem arises from the social science interests of researchers; whereas in the empowering type, the problem emerges from the experience and interests of marginalised groups. In case study 4, for example, the problem was not primarily about how to empower families – they did not own the problem – but how to prove, in terms acceptable to the scientific community, that health visiting was effective. This contrasts with the situation in case study 3, where the problem emerged from the experience of non-abusing mothers, and involved a shift in power relations such that practitioners learned from them. The professionalising type (case study 2) was different again in that professionals identified and pursued the problem. In the organisational type (case study 1), although there may be some negotiation with staff and collaboration, it is the researchers who own the problem.

Differences in terms of problem focus are consistent with differences in ways of thinking about *improvement and involvement*. In the experimental type, improvement is directed towards socially engineered consensus while, at the other end of the typology, empowerment involves a process of negotiation and a recognition that there are likely to be different definitions of what counts as improvement. This is seen not as an obstacle to change but as part of the process of working through change with different groups – in this case, managers, social care workers and a mothers' group. This differs from the professionalising type, where professionals may seek user involvement in the change intervention – such as when piloting patient-centred goal planning – but improvement is defined according to professional criteria. In the organisational type, there may be a concern to produce measurable outcomes, and the assumption is that improvement and involvement are directed towards increasing organisational effectiveness.

The typology used here, however, is only one among several that attempt to provide a framework for thinking about the many issues and dilemmas encountered in action research. To get the best from it, it needs to be used critically and with an open mind. There is no reason to assume that if a particular project does not seem to fit a single type, there is something wrong. It should be used as an aid to thinking and dialogue. If needs be, discard it and move on.

5   Debates and dilemmas

The four types of action research described in Section 4 provide a basis from which to consider three issues – problem identification, generalisability and the relationship between research and action.

Problem identification

Action research is concerned to solve problems in an immediate situation and within a particular setting. As discussed in Section 2, Lewin was insistent that the value of action research lay in its ability to apply the experimental methods of the natural sciences to pressing social problems of the day. For action researchers, the use of the word 'problem' does not necessarily imply that something is wrong – although there may be – but rather that there is a need for change and improvement (Cunningham, 1993). Part of the skill of diagnosing (Figure 1) is to transform what might start out as little more than a feeling that things could be done better into a 'problem' that can be worked on. This was brought out particularly clearly in case studies 3 and 4.

'Problem' is another way of referring to what Lewin called the 'general idea' and, as we saw when considering the cyclic processes of action research (Section 2), the general idea is not fixed, but is subject to modification and reworking in the light of further fact finding and analysis. Eden et al. (1983, p. 13) observe:

> ... the step between feeling some sort of discomfort or dissatisfaction, feeling that there is some problem somewhere, and being able to say 'The problem is such-and-such' is a very big step. In fact quite often we find that if we can say what the problem is we have gone a long way towards solving it. This seems to be true with any kind of problem, whether it be some technically orientated work problem, a relationship problem at home, or anything in between.

Different individuals and groups may also perceive the same situation very differently, and what might be a major problem for one person may be a minor irritation for another. In other words, 'No situation is inherently, "objectively" a problem' (Eden et al., 1983, p. 8).

Action researchers who address the issue of how to bring about change quickly realise that there may be divergent perspectives about what the problem is and who owns it. As East and Robinson found out in an action research study of change in a district health authority:

> Contrary to the usual expectations in the conduct of research, it was not possible to spell out the precise nature of the research problem at the start of the project ... [and] researchers may need to adapt to changing circumstances as the research process unfolds.
>
> (East and Robinson, 1994, pp. 57–58)

They also emphasise the sheer complexity of the task of facilitating change. In their study, they had to address the divergent views of senior managers and senior ward nurses about just where the problems of standards of care originated.

Generalisability

Because action research is essentially problem solving and context-specific, the generalisability of findings may be limited.

> Action researchers, however, do not make claims so much on the grounds of scientific rigour, as in terms of generating findings which are useful and relevant. It is the focus on improvement of practice and on the collaboration between participants to achieve, sustain and learn from such programmes which make it attractive for practitioners.
>
> (Hart and Bond, 1995b, pp. 12–13)

This is not to say that rigour is of no importance in action research – far from it – rather that action researchers have a double responsibility since they need to demonstrate both *rigour* and *relevance*. Action research projects can be seen as similar to qualitative approaches in this respect, as the following comment suggests.

> The idea of sampling from a population of sites in order to generalize to the larger population is simply and obviously unworkable in all but the rarest situations for qualitative researchers, who often take several years to produce an intensive case study of one or a very small number of sites.
>
> (Schofield, 1993, p. 205)

But there are wider issues here too. Bennett, whose collaborative project was discussed in case study 2, pointed to the way in which the findings of the Rivermead team were made available through peer-reviewed journals, so that judgement about generalisability or applicability rests with the readership. Further assessment opportunities in this case were open to those and with those who took up the opportunity to join the training workshops generated by the interest in the published work. Bennett comments:

> I should like to suggest that through discussion of the published work, participation in the training workshops and attempting to introduce patient-centred goal planning, our team has judged the Rivermead model to be generalizable to our own clinical setting. We already share the same theoretical foundation upon which the model has been built, that is our understanding of the therapeutic benefits of structured, patient-centred goals in neurorehabilitation, and the model itself provides us with a framework that we can modify to our own particular setting.
>
> (Bennett, 1998, p. 230)

As Bennett's project showed, one way of looking at generalisability in action research is to ask the question 'To what extent can what has been learned from one project be transferred to another?'. Because this is a very broad question, it encompasses several others, such as 'What kind of evidence is this and what can I make of it?', 'How does the situation I am in differ – or not – from the one in this study?' and 'What might be transferable from one project to another?'. This is how Pat explained it, when writing about what she had taken forward from the 'knowing mothers' project:

> At a personal and professional level, I have been able to transfer the research skills I developed on the course to a new job setting up a post-qualifying framework for a social services department. Adoption of a research and action stance meant that I replicated the process used in the study with the mothers by interviewing potential participants across the country, to collect their views about what they wanted, and to establish amongst them shared ownership of the initiative.
>
> (Bond *et al.*, 1998, p. 121)

Relationship between research and action

This chapter began with Rapoport's concern that one of the dilemmas of action research was that it aimed to be relevant both to the goals of social science and to organisational problem solving. Over a quarter of a century later, such concerns may seem outdated, particularly with the development of practitioner action research. Because of this, some practitioners assume that in undertaking problem-based projects in their own organisations they somehow avoid this particular dilemma. But no research, however practical, can avoid questions of its relationship to bodies of theory and traditions of thought in academic disciplines. Also, as Gill and Johnson noted of management students, those who work in an action research tradition:

> ... will, even if working full time as a manager, probably be stereotyped as an academic – with all that may imply for the successful outcome of the work.
>
> (Gill and Johnson, 1991, p. 61)

The implication is that even insiders to the organisation, in taking on a researcher role, may encounter similar problems to an outsider researcher in terms of the acceptability of findings, and the tensions between, for example, the practical requirements of the organisation and those of a university degree. However, as shown in the action research typology, the relationship between research and action, researcher and client, shifts depending on such things as the nature of the problem, whether the researcher is an outsider or an insider, the nature of collaboration and the learning process emerging from that, as well as on the extent to which the project challenges existing power relations. Even in practitioner action research, the tension between research and action, theory and practice, does not go away. It can, however, generate a productive tension that works to the advantage of all concerned (as in case studies 2 and 3). As Fuller and Petch argue:

> ... research, though not simple or capable of being carried out without technical knowledge, is not as mysterious as all that, and ... it is possible for practitioners, with appropriate support and guidance, to enhance

significantly their understanding of the tasks that they and their colleagues take on in their daily practice. We further suggest that it is possible to attain a productive marriage between the systematic intellectual enquiry which characterizes research and the tough-minded realities of life in social care agencies – indeed, that they are not necessarily opposed. And through such a marriage, we believe, a flow of practitioner research has much to contribute to the developing body of research on social work practice which to date has been largely conducted from outside.

(Fuller and Petch, 1995, p. 4)

Conclusion

The practical focus on problem solving makes action research a particularly attractive option to many practitioners in health and social care. So too does the emphasis on collaborative working found in most of the kinds of action research discussed here. This chapter showed how a range of different approaches to action research is now available. Organisational, professionalising, empowering and experimental action research designs were illustrated and discussed. A typology of action research designs makes clear the contrasting assumptions that can underlie these research designs and highlights important implications which flow from them. Action research brings to the fore some of the complexity of the idea of evidence – the importance of framing and reframing the initial research question, the salience of different kinds of evidence to different kinds of participant.

Acknowledging different definitions of the problem and varieties of evidence and interpretation can be crucial to the process of bringing about change, and action research focuses strongly on how improvement and change come about in a particular setting. Concentrating on single settings does not mean, however, that knowledge transfer is impossible or that questions of rigour in the research design must be abandoned. When it marries rigour with relevance, action research can be a valuable resource for the improvement of practice.

References

Adelman, C. (1993) 'Kurt Lewin and the origins of action research', *Educational Action Research*, Vol. 1, No. 1, pp. 7–24.

Allport, G. W. (1948) 'Foreword', in Lewin, G. W. (ed.) *Resolving Social Conflicts*, pp. vii–xiv, New York, Harper and Brothers.

Barker, W. (1992) 'Health visiting: action research in a controlled environment', *International Journal of Nursing Studies*, Vol. 29, No. 3, pp. 251–9.

Bennett, B. (1998) 'Increasing collaboration within a multidisciplinary team: the early stages of a small action research project', *Journal of Advanced Nursing*, Vol. 7, pp. 227–31.

Bond, M., For Mothers By Mothers Group and Walton, P. (1998) 'Knowing mothers: from practitioner research to self-help and organisational change', *Educational Action Research*, Vol. 6, No. 1, pp. 111–29.

Boutilier, M., Mason, R. and Rootman, I. (1997) 'Community action and reflective practice in health promotion research', *Health Promotion International*, Vol. 12, No. 1, pp. 69–78.

Bowling, A. (1997) *Research Methods in Health*, Buckingham, Open University Press.

Carr, W. and Kemmis, S. (1986) *Becoming Critical: Education, Knowledge and Action Research*, London, Falmer Press.

Collins, D. (1998) *Organisational Change: Sociological Perspectives*, London, Routledge.

Cunningham, I. (1993) 'Interactive holistic research: researching self-managed learning', in Reason, P. (ed.) *Human Inquiry in Action*, pp. 163–81, London, Sage.

East, L. and Robinson, J. (1994) 'Change in process: bringing about change in health care through action research', *Journal of Clinical Nursing*, Vol. 3, pp. 57–61.

Eden, C., Jones, S. and Sims, D. (1983) *Messing About in Problems: An Informal Structured Approach to Their Identification and Management*, Oxford, Pergamon Press.

Fuller, R. and Petch, A. (1995) *Practitioner Research: The Reflexive Social Worker*, Buckingham, Open University Press.

Garside, P. (1998) 'Organisational context for quality: lessons from the fields of organisational development and change management', *Quality in Health Care*, Vol. 7 (supplement), pp. s8–sl5.

Gill, J. and Johnson, P. (1991) *Research Methods for Managers*, London, Paul Chapman.

Hart, E. and Bond, M. (1995a) *Action Research for Health and Social Care: A Guide to Practice*, Buckingham, Open University Press.

Hart, E. and Bond, M. (1995b) 'Developing action research in nursing', *Nurse Researcher*, Vol. 2, No. 3, pp. 4–14.

Jaques, E. (1951) *The Changing Culture of a Factory*, London, Tavistock.

Kemmis, S. *et al.* (1982) *The Action Research Reader*, Australia, Deakin University Press.

Lauri, S. and Sainio, C. (1998) 'Developing the nursing care of breast cancer patients: an action research approach', *Journal of Clinical Nursing*, Vol. 7, pp. 424–32.

Lewin, K. (1948) 'Action research and minority problems', in Lewin, G. (ed.) *Resolving Social Conflicts: Selected Papers on Group Dynamics by Kurt Lewin*, pp. 201–16, New York, Harper and Brothers.

Meyer, J. E. (1993) 'New paradigm research in practice: the trials and tribulations of action research', *Journal of Advanced Nursing*, Vol. 18, pp. 1066–72.

Rapoport, R. N. (1970) 'Three dilemmas in action research', *Human Relations*, Vol. 23, No. 6, pp. 499–513.

Schofield, J. W. (1993) 'Increasing the generalizability of qualitative research', in Hammersley, M. (ed.) *Social Research: Philosophy, Politics and Practice*, pp. 200–25, London, Sage/The Open University (DEH313 Reader).

Shuttleworth, S., Somerton, M. and Vulliamy, D. (1994) *Collaborative Research for Social Change*, Development and Training, University of Hull.

Susman, G. I. and Evered, R. D. (1978) 'An assessment of the scientific merits of action research', *Administrative Science Quarterly*, Vol. 23, pp. 582–603.

Chapter 6
Producing evidence ethically

Maureen A. Eby

Introduction

Even established researchers can sometimes forget that their research proposal contains issues for the participants and/or the researcher themselves that have wider implications for the health, safety and dignity not only of the participants and researcher but also of society at large. In the drive to have that proposal accepted for funding and/or for academic recognition, researchers sometimes fail to think through the implications of their research, especially those implications that impact directly on the well-being of their participants.

This chapter examines research from an ethical perspective. It will identify ethical issues inherent within the research process from the research participant's perspective. It also looks at the process of ethical review and helps locate within professional perspectives how the research participant is protected by examining the ethical issues found within the various research methods discussed earlier in this book.

1   Development of ethics within research

Concern about the potential harm to participants inherent within research designs is not a purely twentieth century phenomenon. During the late nineteenth century, after an era of medical experimentation conducted under the 'ethos of science and medical progress' (Vollmann and Winau, 1996, p. 1445), concern was expressed about the lack of consent obtained in experimental research. In 1898, Albert Neisser, who discovered the bacterium Gonococcus, was fined by the Royal Disciplinary Court for failing to obtain consent from participants in his clinical trials on serum therapy for syphilis prevention at the University of Breslau (now the University of Wrocław, Poland). Neisser injected cell-free serum from patients with syphilis into patients admitted with other medical conditions, who were never told about the experiment or asked for their consent. When these women contracted syphilis, Neisser concluded that his vaccine had not worked and, as the women were mainly prostitutes, he claimed they had contracted syphilis from their work as prostitutes (Vollmann and Winau, 1996).

During the German Third Reich (1933–1945), medical experimentation brought a new dimension to ethical dilemmas in medical research, which has had a lasting effect on human biomedical research today. After the Nuremberg Trials, a code of practice was drawn up, based on the Articles of the Nuremberg Tribunal in 1947, known as the Nuremberg Code (Eby, 1995).

Following World War Two and the Nuremberg Trials, concern was publicly voiced about the protection of participants involved in research. Yet, despite the outcomes of these trials and the development of the Nuremberg Code, research continued often regardless of its outcome on participants. Some 20 years after the Nuremberg Code, the World Medical Association in 1964 adopted the Declaration of Helsinki, revised in 1996 (South Africa), and currently under review (Nicholson, 1999).

The Declaration cites 12 basic principles, which are somewhat similar to the Nuremberg Code's principles with one major exception. The Nuremberg Code gives primacy to the research participant's voluntary, informed consent, while the Declaration of Helsinki states, 'if the physician considers it essential not to obtain informed consent, the specific reasons for this proposal should be stated in the experimental protocol for transmission to the independent committee' (Medical Research Council, 1998, p. 32).

The Declaration of Helsinki does provide for the independent ethical review of biomedical research. It is apparent, however, that the concept of informed consent has been modified from the Nuremberg Code. Under the Declaration of Helsinki, Nuremberg's rigid requirement for respect for persons is softened, and the requirement for informed consent differentiates between therapeutic and non-therapeutic clinical research. Grodin *et al.* (1993, cited in Seidelman, 1996, p. 1465) believe that the Declaration of Helsinki 'undermined the primacy of subject consent in the Nuremberg Code and replaced it with the paternalistic values of the traditional doctor–patient relationship.'

Despite the development of both the Nuremberg Code, published in 1947, and the Declaration of Helsinki nearly 20 years later, research was still being done without regard to the health and well-being of its participants. The literature cites many examples (Krugman *et al.*, 1978; Campbell *et al.*, 1992; LoBiondo-Wood and Haber, 1994; Lock, 1995; Dowd and Wilson, 1995; Nicholson, 1997; Homan, 1998) but two studies stand out as illustrative of the lack of concern and respect for the individuals involved. The Tuskegee syphilis study (1932–1972), characteristic of medical research of its time and in its treatment of informed consent, is described in Box 1 (overleaf).

Fundamental problems with this longitudinal study were the lack of information given to the participants, the lack of adequate treatment, especially after the discovery of penicillin, and the lack of voluntary consent. Even though in some cases consent was nominally obtained, it was based on misinformation and/or failure to inform the participant of the real risks of the research study.

Box 1: Longitudinal case study – Tuskegee syphilis study (1932–1972)

This study by the US Public Health Service based at the Tuskegee Institute, Macon County, Alabama used two groups of black male farm workers to examine the long-term effects of syphilis. One group consisted of individuals who had the disease while the other group was judged to be free of the disease. Over the years, and despite the advent of penicillin which in the 1950s was accepted as the gold standard treatment for syphilis, no treatment was made available to the group with syphilis. In fact, some commentators suggest that efforts were made to keep the group from learning about or even receiving penicillin. The study ended in 1972 after a Congressional investigation, which led to the enactment of legislation establishing institutional review boards or local research ethics committees.

(Source: based on Kampmeier, 1972; Cobb, 1973; Benedek, 1978; LoBiondo-Wood and Haber, 1994; Brawley, 1998)

The second example, which also illustrates this lack of concern and respect for the research participants involved, is Stanley Milgram's *Behavioural Study of Obedience* (1963), described in Box 2.

Box 2: Experimental design – behavioural study of obedience (1963)

Stanley Milgram (1933–1984), investigating the destructiveness of obedience, designed an experiment in which informed subjects – 40 men – administered increasingly higher voltages of electricity to a victim – a white Anglo-Irish male – within a teaching–learning situation; that is, when the victim either gave the wrong response or was unwilling or refused to answer a question, ever-increasing electrical shocks were administered. In reality, the electrical generator was a fake, and the victim, a confederate of the experimenter, was acting out the moans, cries and screams in response to allegedly receiving electrical shocks.

At the end of the experiment, 26 subjects obeyed the commands of the experimenter and administered the highest shock – 450 volts – on the generator even when there was no response from the victim; while 14 subjects broke off the experiment between 300 and 375 volts, after the victim protested and refused to provide further answers. Milgram was surprised by the high number of individuals who were willing to administer what was supposedly a lethal electrical shock, but he did not expect the extreme levels of anxiety exhibited by some of the subjects.

(Source: based on Milgram, 1963)

Box 3: Fundamental ethical principles

The principle of respect for persons

- The duty to respect the rights, autonomy and dignity of other people.

- The duty to promote their well-being and autonomy.

- The duty of truth-full-ness, *honesty* and sincerity (honour = respect), for deceit is *dishonourable*.

(The concept of a person (i.e. a bearer of rights and duties) is the constitutive principle for both law and ethics (and politics).)

The principle of justice

- The duty of universal fairness or equity.

- The duty to treat people as ends, never simply as means to an end.

- The duty to avoid discrimination, abuse or exploitation of people on grounds of race, age, sex, class, gender, or religion.

(The principle of justice requires of us that any personal rule of action we use, should, in principle, be capable of being universalised for all people. For this reason it is sometimes described as the principle of universalisability.)

The principle of beneficence (or non-maleficence)

- The duty to do good and avoid doing harm to others.

- The duty of care, to protect the weak and vulnerable.

- The duty of advocacy: defending the rights of the weak and vulnerable, or incompetent.

(Like the golden rule (do unto others as you would have them do unto you), this principle is sometimes referred to as the principle of reciprocity.)

(Source: Thompson *et al.*, 1994, p. 59)

---

which various health care professional organisations' guidelines and codes are based.

Thinking of these principles when reviewing a research protocol within the health and social care field might raise questions that hitherto had not been apparent. For example, would the researchers in the Tuskegee study still not have treated the research participants with penicillin if they had considered the principles of justice and non-maleficence? Or, based on the principle of respect for autonomy and truthfulness, would the researchers have disclosed to the participants the true nature of their participation in this research study?

Human rights approach

Human rights are claims and demands of individuals or groups that are justified in the eyes of society. Essentially there are five basic human rights as shown in Table 1 (opposite), which also gives examples of when these rights are violated. An ethical review should ensure that the research participants' basic human rights are not violated, which essentially was the basic principle underpinning the Nuremberg Code (1947). Interestingly though, the right to fair treatment and the right to anonymity and confidentiality are not mentioned in the Nuremberg Code – or in the Declaration of Helsinki for that matter.

Using these five basic rights as the framework for an ethical review might raise questions that had not previously been considered. For example, in Milgram's study, the participants' right to self-determination was violated through the deception of the experimental design. The rather impressive electrical generator was an elaborate fake – it could not deliver an electric shock at all. Consequently, the victim had to feign his responses, leading the research participants to believe he was actually being injured to the point that his silence was construed by them as his death.

Questions to ask in an ethical review

The ethical review of research, whether through formal institutional review or by the individual, rests upon a reflective and deliberative interrogation of the researcher's research design and methods based on fundamental ethical principles and approaches. Within health care, the local research ethics committees (LRECs) or the centralised multicentred research ethics committees (MRECs) have a proforma framework that essentially addresses the questions in Box 4.

Box 4: Ethical review of research

Validity of the research (consequence-based)

- How important is the research question?
- Can the research answer the question being asked?

Welfare of the research subject (duty-based)

- What will participating in the research involve?
- Are any risks necessary and acceptable?

Dignity of the research subject (rights-based)

- Will consent be sought?
- Will confidentiality be respected?

(Source: based on Department of Health, 1997, p. 11)

Basic human right	Definition	Examples of violation
Right to self-determination	Based on the ethical principle of respect for persons; people should be treated as autonomous agents who have the freedom to choose without external controls. An autonomous agent is one who is informed about a proposed study and is allowed to choose to participate or not to participate; and research participants have the right to withdraw from a study without penalty Research participants with diminished autonomy are entitled to protection. They are more vulnerable because of age, legal or mental incompetence, terminal illness, or confinement to an institution Justification for use of vulnerable subjects must be provided	A research participant's right to self-determination is violated through the use of coercion, covert data collection and deception Coercion is when an overt threat of harm or excessive reward is presented to ensure compliance Covert data collection is when people become participants and are exposed to research treatments without knowing it Deception is when subjects are actually misinformed about the purpose of the research Potential for violation of the rights to self-determination is greater for research participants with diminished autonomy; they have decreased ability to give informed consent and are vulnerable
Right to privacy and dignity	Based on the principle of respect. Privacy is the freedom of a person to determine the time, extent and circumstances under which private information is shared or withheld from others	Invasion of privacy occurs most frequently during data collection when invasive questions are asked that might result in loss of job, friendships or dignity, or might create embarrassment and mental distress. It also may occur when subjects are unaware that information is being shared with others
Right to anonymity and confidentiality	Based on the principle of respect. Anonymity exists when the subject's identity cannot be linked even by the researcher with his or her individual responses Confidential means that individual identities of research participants will not be linked to the information they provide and will not be publicly divulged	Anonymity is violated when the research participant's responses can be linked with their identity Confidentiality is breached when a researcher, by accident or by direct action, allows an unauthorised person to gain access to study data that contain information about the research participant's identity or responses that create a potentially harmful situation for that participant
Right to fair treatment	Based on the ethical principle of justice, people should be treated fairly and should receive what they are due or owed Fair treatment is equitable selection of research participants and their treatment during the research study. This includes selection of research participants for reasons directly related to the problem studied versus convenience, compromised position, or vulnerability. It also includes fair treatment of research participants during the study including fair distribution of risks and benefits regardless of age, race or socio-economic status	There have been injustices in selecting research participants as a result of social, cultural, racial and gender biases in society Historically, research participants are often from groups of people who were regarded as having less 'social value', poor people, prisoners, slaves, mentally incompetent and dying people. Often research participants were treated carelessly without consideration of physical or psychological harm
Right to protection from discomfort and harm	Based on the ethical principle of beneficence, people must take an active role in promoting good and preventing harm Discomfort and harm can be physical, psychological, social or economic in nature. Levels of harm range from no anticipated effects to temporary discomfort to unusual levels of temporary discomfort to risk of permanent damage to, finally, certainty of permanent damage	A research participant's right to be protected is violated when researchers know in advance that harm, death or disabling injury will occur and thus the benefits do not outweigh the risk

(Source: adapted from LoBiondo-Wood and Haber, 1994, pp. 324–7)

These six questions form an ethical framework based on a consequences, a duties and a rights-based approach to ethics. The questions can
be used to examine research designs, methods and their effects on research
participants. Some people feel this type of proforma framework does not
go far enough in ensuring the protection of the research subject (Eby,
1995; Ashcroft, 1998; Smith, 1999; Sprumont, 1999). For example, will the
research participant be protected from both physical and emotional harm?
Allowing the researcher to calculate the risk may not always be in the best
interest of the research participant. These questions also fail to identify the
hidden social and political pressures underpinning the researcher's
epistemological and ideological basis. Fernando (1989, pp. 250–51, cited
in Patel, 1999, p. 9), drawing upon research into the area of mental health,
suggests:

> ... that the prevailing political context must be taken into account in
> examining the effects of mental health research published in scientific
> journals. ... it is naïve to assume that research on issues involving 'race' is
> value free when conducted in a racist society, within a discipline, such as
> psychiatry, with a powerful racist tradition.

3   Ethical issues within research design

Both the principles and human rights approaches to the ethical review of
research are discussed in this section, which focuses on specific ethical
issues emerging out of the research designs discussed in earlier chapters.
A series of research vignettes will be the focus of discussion. Although
aimed at being representative, they cannot of course cover the complete
range of research methods available. However, the aim of this section is
to highlight some of the major ethical issues found within these
representative examples.

Vignette 1 (opposite) illustrates a pharmaceutical randomised control
trial (RCT), which will provide the evidence needed by a drug company for
establishing a safe and effective dosage range required for drug licensing.
Three crucial aspects of the RCT raise ethical concerns: the process of
randomisation; the intervention itself; and the use of a control group.
Ethical concerns for the process of randomisation relate to the research
participant's consent to enter the trial based on that individual's understanding of what the trial was about.

Research by Kate Featherstone and Jenny Donovan (1998, cited in
Joule, 1998, p. 23) showed that, even though patients could indicate an
understanding of the concept of randomisation, they nevertheless
thought that the doctor had assigned them to a group based on their
own symptoms and medical history. This, as Featherstone indicates, has
'implications for informed consent. Perhaps patients need to be given the
opportunity to explore these issues more fully before consenting to
participation in a trial' (Featherstone, 1998, cited in Joule, 1998, p. 24).

Vignette 1: Randomised controlled trial – protocol for a dose-finding study of G1234 (a new drug) in patients with uncomplicated essential hypertension

This is a single-centre, randomised, double-blind, placebo-controlled trial to evaluate a new drug, G1234, which lowers blood pressure. Animal studies have shown that G1234 is well tolerated to 50 mg/kg/day. Phase I studies of single doses up to 100 mg of G1234 in 12 volunteers showed rapid oral absorption to peak levels in one to two hours and only one volunteer exhibiting a significant drop in blood pressure but without fainting. This proposed study will last nine weeks and is in three stages: Stage 1 – a four-week wash-out period without medications to establish a baseline of the subject's hypertension; Stage 2 – a four-week treatment period consisting of a double-blind placebo-controlled randomised parallel comparison of three different dosages (12.5 mg, 25 mg, 50 mg) and a placebo; and Stage 3 – a one-week wash-out follow-up period without drugs.

Subjects, to be recruited from out-patient clinics, will be aged 18 to 70, with a diagnosis of essential hypertension and with a diastolic blood pressure between 95 and 125 mm Hg at each of the last two visits before the start of Stage 1. After obtaining consent and detailed screening investigations to rule out exclusion criteria, eligible subjects will be withdrawn from their current anti-hypertensive medication and switched to a placebo medication for the wash-out period. After this, subjects will be randomly allocated to 12.5 mg, 25 mg or 50 mg of the drug or to the placebo in Stage 2. Subjects will be assessed at each study visit and if, during the active treatment period, the blood pressure remains uncontrolled, the subject can be withdrawn from the study at the discretion of the investigator.

(Source: based on Department of Health, 1997, pp. 38–39)

In the case of pharmaceutical drug trials, consent to participate from competent adults is required by UK, European and international regulations. In the UK, the Department of Health's *Guidelines to Local Research Ethics Committees* (1991, reprinted in McHale *et al.*, 1997, p. 573) advises that consent be obtained in writing and, in the case of therapeutic research as in Vignette 1, consent should be recorded in the patient's medical record.

Currently, the *ICH Harmonised Tripartite Guidelines for Good Clinical Practice* (ICH, 1996) specify required elements that need to be included in the patient information sheets used to recruit individuals into pharmaceutical drug trials. In line with ICH*, the Scottish Office has produced a set of guidelines for researchers preparing patient information sheets and

---

* International Conference on Harmonisation of Technical Requirements for Registration of Pharmaceuticals for Human Use

consent forms. These guidelines will now become integrated into the MRECs' and Scottish LRECs' process of ethical review of research (Scottish Office, 1999, p. 8). Having reliable and valid information is a corner-stone of autonomy and self-determination but it relies on the principle of truth telling and honesty. However, information is only one aspect of consent. Comprehension of the information is crucial to obtaining consent as is the notion of voluntariness, that is, consent obtained free of coercion and undue influence.

Ethical issues arising from the actual intervention under investigation in an RCT relate to the assessment of risk with regards to the potential benefits to be derived from the actual treatment or drug under study. In Vignette 1, individuals are being asked to consider trying out a new drug that will control their blood pressure presumably as well as, if not better than, their current medication. But, if one of this new drug's side-effects is a 25% increase in the risk of stroke, while uncontrolled high blood pressure has only a 15–20% risk of stroke, the risks of this drug outweigh any possible benefits. Will the researchers be truthful and inform the prospective research participants that these risks exist? Under current guidelines they now must and, clearly, this is one aspect of ethical review that is closely scrutinised.

But this is not quite so clear-cut as it seems for it depends on whether the intervention is therapeutic or non-therapeutic, which relates to the acceptable degree of risk an individual should be allowed to face. For non-therapeutic research, it is generally felt that research participants be exposed to only minimal risk, which is defined as 'a risk of injury or death that is no more than that encountered in daily life' (Smith, 1999, p. 90).

This leads on to one of the most highly contentious aspects of RCTs – the use of a control group receiving a placebo rather than the active treatment or intervention being tested. The basis for the use of placebos is that patients who think they are trying out a new treatment tend to expect and then find an improvement in their condition – this is known as the placebo effect (Elander, 1991; Smith, 1999). In Vignette 1, a research participant could be randomised into the control group and for nine weeks be deprived of any real medication for their high blood pressure. Is that acceptable? This use of a non-treatment or placebo group raised issues of deception in the past since research participants were often not told that randomisation into such a group was possible. Given current guidelines that should no longer happen. The use of a blind study also ameliorates the issue of lying since the doctor does not know whether the research participant is having the active or the placebo treatment.

But even with these current changes, the problems of equity and justice still persist. Should not all research participants have equal access to new and potentially beneficial treatment? On the other hand, the safety and efficacy of new treatments can only be established by testing. Treating any participants carries a risk but it may be justified as part of a trial.

Vignette 2 describes another RCT and, like Vignette 1, there is the issue of consent, randomisation and a control group. But, unlike Vignette 1, the control group is not receiving a placebo or no intervention but rather will remain on the same level of service that currently would be available. The issue for this RCT relates to consent from vulnerable groups, that is, homeless and/or with long-term severe mental illness.

Vignette 2: Randomised controlled trial – social services case management

This study's aim was to evaluate the effectiveness of social services case management for individuals with long-term mental illnesses within the community. Participants were referred from hostels for the homeless, night shelters, GP clinics for homeless people, a city council homelessness unit and local voluntary group homes if, in the opinion of the referrer, the person had a severe, persistent, psychiatric disorder, was homeless or about to become homeless, was not coping, was experiencing social isolation or causing disturbances, and was not already within a case management service. Of the 103 individuals referred, 80 agreed to be randomised after initial assessment. Participants were randomised into the case management group or the control group. The case management group was offered an assessment of need with interventions provided. The control group continued to receive the same level of support as before the study.

(Source: based on Marshall *et al.*, 1995)

There are no references in the published article of this research to issues of consent. However, obtaining consent from such a vulnerable group does require careful thought for the issue is not just about an individual's mental capacity to comprehend the information given but, more importantly, it is about the very form and nature of the explanation given. Arguably, all individuals have the right to self-determination and, as the Department of Health guidelines state, 'the presence of mental disorder does not by itself imply incapacity, nor does detention under the Mental Health Act 1983' (Department of Health, 1991, reprinted in McHale *et al.*, 1997, p. 587). However, balancing this right to self-determination and autonomy is the duty on the researcher not to expose the research participant to harm, either physical or psychological.

Guidelines within health care stress the value of allowing people who cannot consent to participate in research (Royal College of Psychiatrists, 1990; Medical Research Council, 1991; Department of Health, 1991) but with the following safeguards in place (Medical Research Council, 1991, p. 22):

- the research protocol is approved by the LREC
- the individual concerned has not expressed any objections either verbally or through action
- in the case of therapeutic research, participation in the research would be in that individual's best interest

- in the case of non-therapeutic research, participation in the research would be of negligible risk to health and not against the individual's best interest.

But do these safeguards deal with the issue of power and control? There may be covert pressure to participate in the research either to please the researcher, who happens also to be that individual's treating doctor, or because the researcher is in a position to influence outcomes for the individual, that is, obtain further treatment or secure housing or additional benefits (Royal College of Psychiatrists, 1990; Mount *et al.*, 1995, cited in Devereux, 1998). This certainly seems to strengthen the paternalistic position of the researcher, one that inhibits the research participant's self-determination and autonomy. As Devereux continues, 'in my experience patients often consider it their duty to participate in a study or see it as some sort of repayment. They may feel obliged to participate because they think that they are indebted to the caring professions as a result of their illness' (Devereux, 1998, p. 58).

Interviewing shares with RCTs similar concerns about consent, although in Vignette 3 the issues of power and control are made more acute by the fact that the researcher interviewed the women in their own homes. This raises issues of privacy, which it can be argued has been invaded, and betrays a sense of hidden coercion since the mothers would undoubtedly feel indebted to the midwives for the safe delivery of their babies. Again it can be argued that the mothers were also a vulnerable population.

Vignette 3: Interviewing – promoting successful breast feeding among women with low incomes

The aim of this study was to identify factors that promoted or discouraged successful breast feeding in a sample of women with low incomes who delivered at a district general hospital. The community midwives were asked to identify postnatal women who had breast-fed their latest baby at least once and who at booking were identified as receiving state benefits or were aged 16–17 and unemployed. In addition, the researcher scanned all postnatal notes returned to the clinic for filing to ensure no eligible woman was overlooked. Of the 20 eligible women only 15 agreed to participate in the study. The women were interviewed in their homes between 21 and 28 days post-delivery using a semi-structured interview format, which lasted from 2 to 3 hours. These interviews were tape-recorded and then transcribed verbatim by the interviewer. The authors' discussion with colleagues concluded that this research was an audit and thus ethical approval was not needed.

(Source: based on Whelan and Lupton, 1998)

Crucial to this research method is the basic human right to confidentiality and anonymity, which is based on the principles of respect and trust, as well as the right to dignity and privacy, which is based on the principles of beneficence and non-maleficence. Interviewing as a research method depends on the ability of the interviewer to probe and search for the hidden voice within the research respondent before the respondent realises what has been said. As Fontana and Frey (1994, p. 373) state, 'the techniques and tactics of interviewing are really ways of manipulating respondents while treating them as objects or numbers rather than individual human beings.' But interviewing can also leave the researcher in a dilemma especially if during the interview the respondent reveals disturbing or painful information or information about illegal behaviour. Does the researcher break confidentiality to reveal this information?

Confidentiality is a principle found in all professional codes and guidelines related to research. Essentially, disclosure of confidential information requires the consent of the individual unless 'disclosure is required by law or by order of the court' or when disclosure is considered 'necessary in the public interest' (UKCC, 1996, p. 27). However, the British Association of Social Workers' *Code of Ethics for Social Work* (1996, p. 5) states that 'information clearly entrusted for one purpose should not be used for another purpose without sanction.'

The Department of Health's *The Protection and Use of Patient Information* (DoH, 1996) states that sometimes it is defensible to disclose confidential information in the public interest without consent or statutory authority. However, there are no clear guidelines on what exactly constitutes 'in the public interest'. The Public Interest Disclosure Act 1998, para. 43B (HMSO, 1998), which came into force on 2 July 1999, defines a protected disclosure as one made in good faith which the employee reasonably believes relates to one of the following situations.

- A criminal offence has been committed, is being committed or is likely to be committed.
- A person has failed, is failing or is likely to fail to comply with any legal obligation to which he or she is subject.
- A miscarriage of justice has occurred, is occurring or is likely to occur.
- The health or safety of any individual has been, is being or is likely to be endangered.
- The environment has been, is being or is likely to be damaged.
- Information tending to show any matter falling within any one of the preceding paragraphs has been, is being or is likely to be deliberately concealed.

The Protection and Use of Patient Information continues:

Each case must be considered on its merits, the main criterion being whether the release of information to protect the public should prevail over the duty of confidence to the patient. The possible therapeutic consequences for the patient must be considered whatever the outcome.

Decisions will sometimes be finely balanced and may concern matters on which NHS staff find it difficult to make a judgement. Therefore it may be necessary to seek legal or other specialist advice or to wait or seek a court order. It is important not to equate 'the public interest' with what may be 'of interest' to the public.

(Department of Health, 1996, p. 18)

Anonymity or the removal of identifying information also reinforces dignity and respect for people, although often this is a neglected area within research design. In the published article for Vignette 3, the authors include short paragraphs taken from the transcriptions of the audio-tapes. There is no mention in the published article of whether they allowed the respondents to look over or verify the transcriptions of their own interviews. Allowing respondents access to the transcribed interviews enhances dignity and reinforces their autonomy.

These short paragraphs, although not attributed by name, are identified by a number and whether the mother was breast feeding or bottle feeding. In that sense, the authors have maintained anonymity. However, the individual respondents reading through the article could recognise themselves by what they had said. Not knowing that what they said in confidence was going to be published may well have quite an impact on trust. Seeking permission from research participants to include short extracts of what they said in the interview in publications further enhances the trust between researcher and participant.

Vignette 3 also describes the dilemma researchers face between audit and research and whether an ethical review is needed. Audit is about monitoring the services offered to patients and clients. 'Audit seeks to improve practice and treatment and to reduce risk by the systematic review of the process and outcomes of care and treatment and by the evaluation of records and other data' (UKCC, 1996, p. 36) or, as the British Medical Association states, 'Research is concerned with discovering the right thing to do; audit with ensuring that it is done right' (BMA, 1996, p. 5).

The BMA (1996) and the UKCC (1996) have recommended that audit projects do not need to be submitted for ethical review by a research ethics committee but rather that audit committees set up to co-ordinate audit projects should consider the ethical issues that arise from audit such as confidentiality, anonymity, consent to use patient/client's records, and the scientific validity of the proposed audit methodology. Avoiding ethical review by LRECs does not remove the researcher's obligation to ensure that the research participants are not exposed to unacceptable risks and do derive some benefits from co-operating in the research.

Action research 'is simply a form of self-reflective enquiry undertaken by participants in social situations in order to improve the rationality and justice of their own practices, their understanding of these practices, and the situations in which the practices are carried out' (Carr and Kemmis, 1986, p. 162; see also Chapter 5 of this book). Action research in Vignette 4 aims to empower the participants, which appears to have been the goal of the day care centre for people with learning difficulties. In this action research, the researcher and participants became partners, although whether they are equal partners is questionable. In this case, the participants involved individuals with learning difficulties, a vulnerable group. This raises the issue of consent – first, to whom are the participants giving their consent and, second, to what have the participants consented (Williams, 1995)?

Vignette 4: Action research – day care on the move

This project focused on a day care centre for adults with learning difficulties and aimed to change the culture of the centre from care management and principled contracting to one of user involvement and choice through participative action research. Individuals with learning difficulties and the day care centre staff, using the Scottish Human Services package *Changeover*, became co-researchers to create shared and usable knowledge that aimed to transform the culture of the day centre. The techniques used to facilitate the change were group discussion, brainstorming, SWOT analyses, and reflective discussion. The outcomes of these activities were the development of network groups and a self-advocacy group, which has created a new discourse that challenges traditional disablist discourse.

(Source: based on Baldwin, 1997)

Were these participants giving consent to the researcher – the individual charged with implementing the changeover from case management to user choice – or were they consenting to the organisation itself – the day care centre – to act as volunteers in this changeover process? And what exactly were they consenting to? Was it to continue to participate in the day care centre? Or were they actually consenting to the change itself, that is, instead of case management, the participants were consenting to the changeover to user involvement and choice?

As Williams (1995, p. 52) suggests, 'action researchers normally try to facilitate change in *others*. In "helping", "facilitating" and "emancipating", one runs the risk of being labelled patronising.' Change itself also brings the element of fear of the unknown. In this case, fear of the day care centre closing could well have prompted the participants to consent. Given the complexities found within consent in action research, the scope for deception in these circumstances raises many questions regarding power and control.

Confidentiality also becomes an issue if the participants are co-researchers and partners. Who, then, makes decisions about what is revealed or not and to whom it is revealed? As Williams (1995, p. 55) points out:

> ... ideas about democracy and egalitarianism in some ways sit uneasily with ideas about the responsibility of researchers to protect and

maintain the integrity of research participants. If the so called 'co-researchers' had equal control over the research, then confidentiality would be a matter of a collective agreement on the part of all co-researchers (including 'the researcher') to respect the sensitivities of all.

Vignette 5 raises three kinds of issues. The first concerns the open-ended nature of qualitative research, which is often started without the researcher knowing exactly what will be found. This makes it very difficult for researchers to seek ethical approval from ethics committees in advance of the research being done. Similarly, it is difficult for research participants to be forewarned about what the researcher is exactly looking for, which makes informed consent an impossible task. Usually, it is not until researchers are well into analysing the data after leaving the research location that they know what the data are saying. Some researchers tackle this problem by offering the research participants the opportunity to read and comment on the draft research publication. But should the researcher allow those studied to rewrite the research findings? Vignette 5 poses this problem in its most extreme form. If Bowler had warned the staff of her growing interest in racist stereotypes and discriminatory practices then presumably the staff would have modified and changed their expressed views and practices. If she had offered editorial control over the published results then it is unlikely this study would have been published.

Vignette 5: Evaluation – ethnographic research in an obstetrics unit

Isobel Bowler spent three months observing activities in a maternity hospital and recording what she saw and heard. She also held in-depth interviews with midwives, obstetricians and mothers. Her particular interest was in how South Asian mothers were thought about, spoken about and treated by staff. Her findings present a picture of white staff holding racist stereotypes about South Asian women and of poor midwifery and obstetrics practice for South Asian mothers in comparison with white mothers. It is not clear how Bowler explained the purpose of her research to the staff or to the mothers. But, given the results, it seems reasonable to assume she did not forewarn the staff she was particularly interested in their racism. The hospital concerned was made anonymous in the published research, but there must have been many people who knew where Bowler had done her research, including the people who are quoted extensively in the published article.

(Source: based on Bowler, 1993)

The second issue raised by Bowler's study is about striking a balance between the rights of those studied to confidentiality, privacy and honesty versus the benefits to be derived from being reticent about the purpose of the research and then breaching privacy by publishing the results in order to draw attention to institutional racism within obstetric care.

The third issue concerns the most effective means to combat racism. Would it have been more effective to have abandoned the research to draw attention to institutional racism within the hospital concerned; perhaps to have the issue successfully dealt with locally? Or was it more effective to do as Bowler actually did, which was to collude with racist practice for the duration of the research in order to produce evidence that might be used to confront racism in midwifery more generally?

It should be obvious that too enthusiastic an adherence to the values of privacy, confidentiality and non-deceptive research would make abuse, malpractice and discrimination no-go areas for researchers. Much the same might be said for the value of doing no harm to the people studied, if they engage in racial or sexual discrimination, or unlawful or unprofessional activities. Looking again at the deception practised by Milgram (Section 1), it is perhaps worth suggesting that, although his research would not be passed by a research ethics committee today, the study has been enormously valuable in demonstrating the power of obedience. Among other things, it is frequently cited in discussions of research ethics to illustrate how easy it is for researchers to persuade people to consent to research in which they really do not want to be involved.

Conclusion

This chapter focused on the process of producing evidence ethically. Whether as a user of research, a research participant, a reader of research for work or professional development, or a researcher designing and carrying out research, ethical review is a fundamental part of the research process. Considering how the evidence was obtained is an important step in its evaluation. Without ethical guidelines, informed by explicit ethical principles, there would be no shared basis on which to judge the appropriateness of the research strategy. The desire to construct a tight research design and produce clear findings that will be of future value to other service-users may often be in conflict with individuals' rights to respect and dignity. A very respectful piece of research may be ethically sound and a positive experience for participants, but it may nevertheless fail to provide any useful contributions to knowledge. Ultimately, the issues are value-based. The challenge, for researchers and practitioners alike, is to judge research in terms of how well it keeps its balance – between rigour and respect. In other words, how far it succeeds in producing evidence ethically.

References

Ashcroft, R. (1998) 'One year on: LRECs & MRECs in the West Country', *Bulletin of Medical Ethics*, No. 143, November, pp. 8–11.

Association of Directors of Social Services Research Group (1996) *Guidelines for Researchers Wanting Support from the ADSS Research Group*, Winchester, Hampshire County Council.

Baldwin, M. (1997) 'Day care on the move: learning from a participative action research project at a day centre for people with learning difficulties', *British Journal of Social Work*, Vol. 27, No. 6, December, pp. 951–58.

Baumrind, D. (1964) 'Some thoughts on ethics of research: after reading Milgram's behavioural study of obedience', *American Psychologist*, Vol. 19, pp. 421–23.

Benedek, T. (1978) 'The Tuskegee study of syphilis: analysis of moral versus methodologic aspects', *Journal of Chronic Disease*, Vol. 31, No. 1, pp. 35–50.

Bowler, I. (1993) ' "They're not the same as us": midwives' stereotypes of South Asian descent maternity patients', *Sociology of Health and Illness*, Vol. 15, No. 2, pp. 157–78.

Brawley, O. (1998) 'The study of untreated syphilis in the negro male', *International Journal of Radiation Oncology Biological Physics*, Vol. 40, No. 1, pp. 5–8.

Brechin, A., Brown, H. and Eby, M.A. (eds) (2000) *Critical Practice in Health and Social Care*, London, Sage (K302 Book 1).

British Association of Social Workers (1996) *The Code of Ethics for Social Work*, Birmingham, BASW.

British Medical Association (1996) *Ethical Issues in Clinical Audit*, London, BMA.

Campbell, A., Gillett, G. and Jones, G. (1992) *Practical Medical Ethics*, Auckland, New Zealand, Oxford University Press.

Carr, W. and Kemmis, S. (1986) *Becoming Critical: Education, Knowledge and Action Research*, London, The Falmer Press.

Cobb, W. (1973) 'Briefs: The Tuskegee syphilis study', *Journal of the National Medical Association*, Vol. 65, No. 4, pp. 345–48.

Department of Health (1991) *Guidelines to Local Research Ethics Committees*, London, Department of Health, reprinted in McHale *et al.* (1997), pp. 568–97.

Department of Health (1996) *The Protection and Use of Patient Information*, 7 March, London, Department of Health.

Department of Health (1997) *Briefing Pack for Research Ethics Committee Members*, London, Department of Health.

Devereux, J. (1998) 'A personal experience of research', *Nursing Times*, Vol. 94, No. 9, 4 March, pp. 57–58.

Dowd, S. and Wilson, B. (1995) 'Informed patient consent: a historical perspective', *Radiologic Technology*, Vol. 67, No. 2, pp. 119–24.

Eby, M. (1994) *The Law and Ethics of General Practice*, Beckenham, Kent, Publishing Initiatives.

Eby, M. (1995) 'Ethical issues in nursing research: the wider picture', *Nurse Researcher*, Vol. 3, No. 1, September, pp. 5–13.

Elander, G. (1991) 'Ethical conflicts in placebo treatment', *Journal of Advanced Nursing*, Vol. 16, pp. 947–51.

Featherstone, K. and Donovan, J. (1998) 'Random allocation or allocation at random? Patients' perspectives of participation in a randomised controlled trial', *British Medical Journal*, Vol. 317, pp. 1177–80.

Fernando, S. (1989) 'Schizophrenia in ethnic minorities', *Psychiatric Bulletin*, Vol. 13, pp. 250–51.

Fontana, A. and Frey, J. (1994) 'Interviewing', in Denzin, N. and Lincoln, Y. (eds) *Handbook of Qualitative Research*, pp. 361–76, London, Sage.

Grbich, C. (1999) *Qualitative Research in Health*, London, Sage.

Grodin, M., Annas, G. and Glantz, L. (1993) 'Medicine and human rights: a proposal for international action', *Hastings Center Report*, Vol. 23, pp. 8–12.

Gross, R. (1996) *Psychology: The Science of Mind and Behaviour* (3rd edn), London, Hodder and Stoughton.

Her Majesty's Stationery Office (HMSO) (1998) *Public Interest Disclosure Act 1998*, London, HMSO. (http://www.hmso.gov.uk/acts/acts1998/19980023.htm#aofs – accessed 26 March 1999)

Homan, R. (1998) 'The effects of social research', in Marsh, I. (ed.) *Classic and Contemporary Readings in Sociology*, pp. 350–55, Harlow, Longman.

Hornsby-Smith, M. (1993) 'Gaining access', in Gilbert, N. (ed.) *Researching Social Life*, pp. 52–67, London, Sage.

International Conference on Harmonisation of Technical Requirements for Registration of Pharmaceuticals for Human Use (ICH) (1996) *ICH Harmonised Tripartite Guidelines for Good Clinical Practice*, Geneva, ICH Secretariat.

Joule, N. (1998) '50 years of clinical trials: past, present and future', *Bulletin of Medical Ethics*, No. 142, October, pp. 22–24.

Kampmeier, R. (1972) 'The Tuskegee study of untreated syphilis', *Southern Medical Journal*, Vol. 65, No. 10, October, pp. 1247–51.

Krugman, S., Friedman, H. and Lattimer, C. (1978) 'Hepatitis A and B: serologic survey of various population groups', *The American Journal of the Medical Sciences*, Vol. 275, No. 3, May–June, pp. 249–55.

LoBiondo-Wood, G. and Haber, J. (1994) *Nursing Research* (3rd edn), St Louis, Missouri, Mosby.

Lock, S. (1995) 'Research ethics – a brief historical review to 1965', *Journal of Internal Medicine*, Vol. 238, pp. 513–20.

Marshall, M., Lockwood, A. and Garth, D. (1995) 'Social services case-management for long-term mental disorders: a randomised controlled trial', *The Lancet*, Vol. 345, 18 February, pp. 409–12.

McHale, J., Fox, M. and Murphy, J. (1997) *Health Care Law: Text and Materials*, London, Sweet and Maxwell.

Medical Research Council (1991) *The Ethical Conduct of Research on the Mentally Incapacitated*, MRC Ethics Series, London, MRC.

Medical Research Council (1998) *MRC Guidelines for Good Clinical Practice in Clinical Trials*, MRC Clinical Trials Series, London, MRC.

Milgram, S. (1963) 'Behavioural study of obedience', *Journal of Abnormal and Social Psychology*, Vol. 67, No. 4, pp. 371–78.

Milgram, S. (1974) *Obedience to Authority*, New York, Harper and Row.

Mount, B., Cohen, R., Macdonald, N. *et al.* (1995) 'Ethical issues in palliative care research revisited', *Palliative Medicine*, Vol. 9, No. 2, pp. 165–70.

Nicholson, R. (1997) 'Ethics and the use of ionising radiation in research on humans', *Bulletin of Medical Ethics*, No. 132, October, pp. 13–22.

Nicholson, R. (1999) 'Helsinki Declaration revising continues', *Bulletin of Medical Ethics*, No. 146, March, pp. 3–5.

Parker, B. (1994) 'Research ethics committees', in Tschudin, V. (ed.) *Ethics: Education and Research*, pp. 72–112, Harrow, Scutari Press.

Patel, N. (1999) *Getting the Evidence: Guidelines for Ethical Mental Health Research Involving Issues of 'Race', Ethnicity and Culture*, London, Mind Publications.

Rowson, R. (1990) *An Introduction to Ethics for Nurses*, London, Scutari Press.

Royal College of Psychiatrists (1990) 'Guidelines for psychiatric research involving human subjects', *Psychiatric Bulletin*, Vol. 14, p. 49, reprinted in McHale *et al.* (1997), pp. 587–89.

Scottish Office (1999) 'Guidelines for researchers: patient information sheet and consent form', *Bulletin of Medical Ethics*, No. 148, May, pp. 8–12.

Seidelman, W. (1996) 'Nuremberg lamentation: for the forgotten victims of medical science', *British Medical Journal*, Vol. 313, 7 December, pp. 1463–67.

Smith, T. (1999) *Ethics in Medical Research*, Cambridge, Cambridge University Press.

Sprumont, D. (1999) 'Legal protection of human research subjects in Europe', *European Journal of Health Law*, Vol. 6, No. 1, March, pp. 25–43.

Thompson, I., Melia, K. and Boyd, K. (1994) *Nursing Ethics* (3rd edn), Edinburgh, Churchill Livingstone.

Tierney, A. (1995) 'The role of research ethics committees', *Nurse Researcher*, Vol. 3, No. 1, September, pp. 43–52.

United Kingdom Central Council for Nursing, Midwifery and Health Visiting (UKCC) (1996) *Guidelines for Professional Practice*, London, UKCC.

Vollmann, J. and Winau, R. (1996) 'Informed consent in human experimentation before the Nuremberg code', *British Medical Journal*, Vol. 313, 7 December, 1445–47.

Whelan, A. and Lupton, P. (1998) 'Promoting successful breast feeding among women with a low income', *Midwifery*, Vol. 14, pp. 94–100.

Williams, A. (1995) 'Ethics and action research', *Nurse Researcher*, Vol. 2, No. 3, March, pp. 49–59.

Part 2
Putting Research into Practice

Chapter 7
Research and practice: making a difference

Gill Needham

Introduction

> ... research is crucial to midwifery, so that we can ensure that we are giving the best possible care.
>
> ... if we want to give women more choice then we have to give up-to-date, research-based information.
>
> We should be able to learn more about research, more easily. But we can't, we're stuck. You know, we apply for a course, and you have to fight with lots of other people, and you can never get time off work.
>
> The research and knowledge wouldn't be any good without the experience, but the experience wouldn't be any good without the other two.
>
> You see the word research frightens a lot of people, doesn't it? How you are going to get it across is very difficult. It doesn't matter what way you present it, some people are going to be frightened of the changes that are going on. It's just very difficult.
>
> (Meah *et al.*, 1996, pp. 75–76)

These statements were made by a group of midwives in North West England but they could just as well have come from any group of practitioners. They reflect the conflict between a real enthusiasm for practice development and evidence-based practice on the one hand and pressures of time and the complex challenge of changing practice on the other.

Whose responsibility is it to communicate and implement research? Should researchers be held responsible for ensuring that the results of their work are incorporated into day-to-day professional practice? Is it an organisational responsibility for providers of health and social care and, if it is, who in the social services department, the trust or the primary care team should do this and how? Or is it perhaps the responsibility of individual practitioners to keep up to date with the latest evidence in their field and change their practice accordingly? There are no straightforward answers. This chapter will explore some of the barriers to getting research into practice and strategies that can be used to overcome them and reflect on what can be learned from some of the successes and failures.

From time to time we will also draw on two stories – one is a local project and the other a series of national policy initiatives. The fact that both of these case studies are drawn predominantly from health care reflects the resources invested in this kind of work by the NHS in the early 1990s. Social work and social care are going in a similar direction, although with considerably fewer resources and sometimes with more complex issues to address.

1   Barriers to evidence-based practice

In the story told in Box 1, why was there such a variation between the three trusts in Buckinghamshire? And why were there so many unnecessary D&Cs?

Variations in practice between geographical areas, individual hospitals or individual consultants are common. They are usually identified, as in this example, through routinely produced data. While some variations may reflect local policy developed to meet specific local needs, in many cases they are simply a function of individual clinician preference. Is this acceptable? The argument in its defence is that of clinician autonomy and clinical freedom. The medical profession has always protected the rights of individual clinicians to make autonomous decisions.

Women in Buckinghamshire were not alone in being subjected to inappropriate rates of D&C, despite the fact that the evidence summarised in the review article had been around for some time. This forms part of a problem that has become known as the 'research–practice gap'.

The gap between research and practice in health and social care is well documented. Many writers point out that, despite campaigns by government departments and professional bodies to promote evidence-based practice, the rate of change is slow. Hicks and Hennessy (1997), for example, writing about nursing, suggest that nursing practice 'continues to be essentially ritualistic', while Cheetham (1994), reviewing the experience of the Social Work Research Centre at Stirling, describes the frustration experienced by researchers at the 'somewhat tenuous relationship between research and practice'.

Hicks and Hennessy (1997, p. 596) suggest two main reasons:

> In essence it would appear that the problem is dually determined, being caused at the one level by a shortfall in high-quality published research that has the capacity to alter practice (Smith, 1994) and, at the other, by the failure of that research which does exist to inform practitioners and their procedures.

The points are not so very different from the midwives' comments in the introduction to this chapter and we shall examine each of them in turn.

Box 1: D&C in Buckinghamshire – Part 1

In 1993 a review article was published in the medical press (Coulter *et al.*, 1993), which claimed that many young women were having unnecessary surgery. The operation in question was the dilatation of the uterine cervix and curettage of the uterus (known as D&C) and the most common reason for doing this in younger women was menorrhagia (heavy periods). The authors pointed out that the rates of D&C had declined dramatically in the USA while UK rates remained stable (in 1989 to 1990 the rate was 71.1 per 10,000 women in England compared with only 10.8 per 10,000 in the USA). Although a D&C is an investigative procedure (sampling the lining of the womb to check for cancer cells), it had at one time been thought to have therapeutic value too. It was now also being superseded as an investigative procedure by far less invasive methods that can be done in out-patients or in the GP's surgery. The authors recommended that D&C should not be done on women under 40 for heavy periods (because cancer of the uterus in this age group is extremely rare and D&C carries a risk of complications).

Before the publication of this article, public health specialists in Buckinghamshire had been studying information from the three local hospital trusts about the numbers of different surgical procedures in the previous year.

D&C was near the top of the list of most common procedures but the degree of variation between the numbers of D&Cs in the three localities (after standardising the figures to reflect the population) was rather surprising.

The table below shows a marked difference in the frequency of these operations, depending on where the women lived in the county. It shows the numbers of elective D&C operations and the standardised admission ratios (SAR) in women aged 15 to 39 in Buckinghamshire in 1992–3.

	Area A		Area B		Area C	
	No.	SAR	No.	SAR	No.	SAR
1992/3	89	84	124	66	221	159

The table revealed that a woman under 40 living in locality C was more than twice as likely to have a D&C than one living in locality B. Identifying this variation in practice inevitably raised the question 'How many D&Cs would be appropriate?' This question was partially answered by the review article which, summarising the most up-to-date evidence, suggested 'none for heavy periods in women under 40'.

(Source: table adapted from Holton and Needham, 1995, p. 20)

Not enough high-quality research

What do Hicks and Hennessy mean by 'a shortfall in high-quality published research that has the capacity to alter practice'? In many areas of practice, professionals have little choice other than to be guided by their training, evidence from their own experience and 'custom and practice' in their team or organisation because there have been few relevant studies. The problem is more marked in social care where in 1992 a systematic review of studies of the effectiveness of social work interventions found only 23 experimental and 14 quasi-experimental studies. One author notes:

> Even if the number of studies identified were doubled or trebled, it would represent a worrying dearth of concern with the results of the activities of some 39,600 UK social workers (not to mention 42,900 home help, community support, day and residential care workers).
>
> (MacDonald, 1996, p. 39)

Many studies in health and social care are small scale. They may offer helpful and thought-provoking challenges to practice but they can also be of poor quality with inadequate sample sizes or flawed methodology – often reflecting inadequate funding, training and support. Some may be methodologically very sound but difficult to implement in practice. Another key aspect of quality in research therefore is *relevance*. To what extent does research really address the questions practitioners and users need to have answered?

In the NHS, where huge sums have long been invested in research (£435 million a year), the lack of any strategic framework until 1995 meant that there was no formal mechanism for practitioners or users to draw attention to significant knowledge gaps and influence the research agenda. This is gradually being addressed within the NHS R&D Strategy. Similar concerns about a lack of framework for research in the personal social services led to the establishment of independent review (Independent Review Group, 1994).

Failure to implement high-quality research

The other side of the coin is high-quality research that has clear and unambiguous implications for practice but fails to effect any change. Not only does this represent a depressing waste of resources but also, at best, patients and clients are not being offered the best possible care and, at worst, they are experiencing unnecessary suffering. One example has already been given – women having unnecessary D&Cs. For many years children were almost routinely referred for tonsillectomy, despite the lack of any evidence of benefit. More recently, systematic reviews (University of Leeds, 1992) have suggested that inserting grommets into the ears of children with glue ear is unnecessary for all but the most severe of cases.

In these examples patients have been subjected to surgical risk where evidence suggests little benefit. Even more worrying are the examples of people not receiving potentially beneficial treatments. A review by Antman *et al.* (1992) showed that by 1975 there was clear evidence from randomised controlled trials that giving patients who have just had heart attacks clot-busting drugs would reduce mortality by 50%. However, medical textbooks did not begin to recommend routine use of this treatment until the late 1980s. Similarly, inquiries after child abuse cases have criticised social workers for failing to take sufficient account of relevant research (Munro, 1998).

Why is there delay (and in some cases total failure) to integrate research evidence into practice? Box 2 is a brief summary of the many reasons suggested in the literature.

Box 2: Reasons cited for the research–practice gap

Some reasons are about *the ways in which research is communicated*

- Research findings tend to be published in 'academic' or 'obscure' journals which are read by academics rather than practitioners.

- Many health care professionals and the majority of social workers have poor access to specialist libraries and sources of information.

- Where practitioners work in semi-isolation (in the community or primary care) there is less chance of messages from new research being disseminated by person-to-person communication.

- Information overload – the sheer weight of new information being produced.

- When research findings reach and are read by practitioners they are not sufficiently accessible to be understood and valued.

While other reasons are *to do with the practitioners themselves* – lack of skills or confidence, pressure of time and attitudes to research

- Practitioners have little time for professional reading.

- They may lack the time and the skill to sift out the relevant and useful information from the rest.

- Practitioners do not have the skills to critically appraise the papers they read – i.e. to assess their quality and relevance to their practice.

- Practitioners are threatened by challenges to their practice, particularly by researchers.

- Research is not valued. Hicks and colleagues studied attitudes to research in multidisciplinary primary health care teams and found that:

  ... those health carers studied perceived research to be neither important nor central to their role.

  (Hicks *et al.*, 1996, p. 1040)

- Research findings may conflict with long-held beliefs and/or experience of the practitioner. For example, if a practitioner has seen a particular intervention have a drastic effect on one patient or client that experience will always outweigh any research evidence.

- Research findings may seem not to apply to specific individual patients.

- Practitioners cannot see how the suggested change in practice will benefit their patients or clients. They are unlikely to make the investment in time and 'pain' to change their practice without any clear incentive.

- Practitioners may have no clear idea of what they are achieving, and hence may be unable to recognise whether or not research on effective practice is relevant to them.

- Researchers and practitioners 'inhabit different worlds' and speak different languages.

Having considered some of the major barriers to the use of research findings in practice, we now turn to strategies to overcome them and return to the story of D&C in Buckinghamshire (Box 3).

2   Strategies

Box 3: D&C in Buckinghamshire – Part 2

The release of the information about rates of D&C caused some consternation, although the three localities were not identified. A GRiP (Getting Research into Practice) project was set up to try to translate the evidence on D&C into practice across the county. The Local Medical Committee (which represents all GPs) nominated three GPs, one from each locality, to form part of the project team with the public health specialists. An exhaustive literature search served to confirm the message of the review. The team quickly realised that the important question was not 'How can we reduce unnecessary D&C?' but rather, 'What is the best treatment we can offer to women in Bucks who suffer from heavy periods?' and then, having defined that 'best practice', the challenge would be to implement it.

The evidence suggested that women who have heavy periods should generally be managed in primary care, with the GP taking a lead. It seems that too many women had been unnecessarily referred to gynaecologists and then found themselves on a conveyor belt to D&C and then sometimes to hysterectomy. Instead they should be offered a choice of medical treatments, with surgical options as a last resort.

The GRiP team set out to translate the evidence from the literature into some kind of template for best practice – a 'clinical guideline' to be used by GPs (and to a lesser extent by the consultant gynaecologists) in discussion with their women patients. If it were to stand any chance of success the content would have to be carefully negotiated between the GPs and the consultants. The initial reactions from the consultants reflected many of the attitudes listed above – feeling threatened and challenged, questioning the research evidence and the statistics.

The team agreed that it would be the GPs who would 'negotiate' directly with the consultants as they had more credibility as clinicians (and power as fund-holders) than the health authority staff. It was also going to be difficult to get agreement about best practice between the consultants themselves (hardly surprising, considering the practice variation already identified). Painstakingly, a guideline was developed, adapted, discussed and adapted until it was acceptable to GPs and gynaecologists alike.

Improving the communication of research findings

Given the pressures on practitioners, it is hardly surprising that, when asked how they like to read about research findings, they express a preference for easy-to-read summaries with clear messages about implications for practice (Luker and Kenrick, 1995). The major response to this from the organisations concerned with encouraging evidence-based practice has been to promote two kinds of summary of research results:

- systematic reviews (and meta-analyses)

and

- clinical guidelines.

We are all familiar with *reviews* – articles or publications which bring several studies together and provide some kind of summary. They can take many forms – textbooks, editorial articles, specialist review journals and newspaper articles. Reviews can help busy practitioners keep up to date with new research. Unfortunately, reviews can be misleading if they have not been done systematically. This is particularly important if a review of studies of *effectiveness* is to be used as the basis for a decision about a service or a treatment. A *systematic review* uses a structured and clearly described method to try to achieve an unbiased conclusion. The author of a systematic review should go through a number of steps.

1 Define precisely the question the review is addressing.
2 Search as exhaustively as possible for all studies that address the question.
3 Assess the quality of those studies using predefined criteria.
4 Exclude studies that fail to meet the criteria.
5 Provide an overview of the results of the included studies.
6 Interpret those results in terms of implications for practice.

When searching for studies to include, it is important for the systematic reviewer to try to track down unpublished as well as published studies. If a study suggesting that a new expensive wonder drug offers no advantage over the cheaper standard treatment (or, worse, is potentially harmful) remains unpublished while several positive studies are published, it is vital for the reviewer to include both. However, studies with neutral or negative results tend not to be published. The researchers may not submit them in the first place or journal editors may reject them as they are not considered 'interesting'. This results in what is called 'publication bias'.

Here a Dutch reviewer describes his experience of systematically reviewing randomised controlled trials (RCTs) on homeopathy:

> It is a real enterprise that takes its toll in blood, sweat and tears ... Helped by alternative researchers, my colleagues and I turned many libraries upside down to get a collection of 107 controlled trials (published before May, 1991). Medline* yielded only 18 publications. Checking the references and the references of the references increased the number to 30, still not more than 28%. For homeopathy, other sources such as congress reports and dissertations (from Germany and France) were more fruitful.
>
> Most (61%) of the trials that we could find on homeopathy were published in languages other than English. We graded all trials for their methodological quality on a scale of 0 to 100; 16 scored 60 or more points. Only three of the better publications were in English.
>
> (Knipschild, 1995, p. 14)

While systematic reviews are most common in health care, they are becoming increasingly so in social care. A project at the University of Salford was set up in 1998 to explore the feasibility of systematic reviews of research literature on effectiveness and outcomes in social care for adults (see the Appendix). The first area to be systematically reviewed as part of the Salford project was rehabilitation in mental health.

Where several RCTs on a particular topic have used precisely the same methodology, the results can be statistically combined using a technique called *meta-analysis* to give an overall summary result. This is particularly useful where several studies have been done that are *individually* too small to give convincing results. Combining these results through meta-analysis means that important conclusions can be drawn. In 1972 the report of an

---

* A database of medical literature

RCT of giving corticosteroids to women who were expected to deliver their babies prematurely was published. The results demonstrated that this inexpensive course of treatment reduced respiratory distress and hence the likelihood of the babies dying. Between 1972 and 1991 seven more trials were reported, all of which were too small for their results to be used with confidence. In 1989 a systematic review and meta-analysis summarised the results of all the trials and showed conclusively that the treatment is effective.

While systematic reviews bring together the evidence on a topic and make recommendations for practice, *clinical guidelines* (often based on systematic reviews) take the synthesis and interpretation of the evidence one stage further. Clinical guidelines bring together evidence from research, professional and user perspectives and relevant information about the local organisation of care to provide recommendations for good practice. They are:

> Systematically developed statements to assist practitioner and patient decisions about appropriate health care for specific clinical circumstances.
>
> (Mann, 1996)

The format and presentation of guidelines vary considerably. The Buckinghamshire guideline, for example, was presented as a detailed algorithm (or flow diagram) – others may not use diagrams at all. They can vary in size from an A4 sheet to a small book.

While guidelines are often based on the results of systematic reviews, their effectiveness in helping to change practice has itself been systematically reviewed, as Box 4 shows.

Box 4: Do guidelines work?

In 1994 a systematic review addressed the question 'Can guidelines be used to improve clinical practice?' The authors identified 91 studies from a variety of clinical settings and they concluded that:

- introducing guidelines can both change clinical practice and affect patient outcome

- ways in which the guidelines are developed and implemented will affect their success

- the reason for developing them needs to be clear

- they should be developed locally, taking account of local circumstances (nationally produced guidelines can be a useful source of evidence but it is important to avoid the 'not invented here' barrier)

- dissemination through active educational interventions and implementation through patient-specific reminder systems increase the chance of success.

(Source: adapted from Nuffield Institute for Health, 1994, p. 1)

The NHS has invested considerably in disseminating systematic reviews and guidelines to practitioners to help to improve the take-up of research results. Major initiatives include the UK Cochrane Centre (part of the Cochrane Collaboration – an international network of people dedicated to doing systematic reviews) and the NHS Centre for Reviews and Dissemination, whose role is to disseminate reviews to practitioners and users (including the publication of *Effective Health Care Bulletins*). These initiatives are described more fully in the Appendix. Similarly, one of the functions of the National Institute for Clinical Excellence (NICE) is to review and communicate guidelines. These efforts are based on the assumption that synthesised and summarised research findings, disseminated appropriately, will lead to changes in practice.

The Buckinghamshire GRiP experience, focused as it was on GPs, supports the above review's conclusion about the importance of local ownership. The process of developing the guidelines was open and systematic and attempts were made to keep relevant groups informed. In retrospect, however, the definition of stakeholders should have been broader. Other professionals, particularly practice nurses and community pharmacists, could have been involved in the development process as could patient representatives.

Helping people change practice

Box 5: D&C in Buckinghamshire – Part 3

Copies of the guideline incorporating the Local Medical Committee endorsement were posted with an explanatory letter to all GPs in the county. The GRiP project team felt an enormous sense of achievement. They did not realise at that time that the process of *implementation* had not yet even begun.

Getting research into practice requires both the *communication*, or what is often called *dissemination*, of results and the *implementation* of findings through changes to practice. Dissemination of results on its own is not sufficient to produce change. (In practice, however, the terms *dissemination* and *implementation* are often used loosely and interchangeably.) In fact, the GRiP team had a range of strategies from which to choose. There is some evidence about the effectiveness of these (mainly from systematic reviews in the field of medicine). The strategies and the evidence are summarised in Table 1.

Table 1   **Strategies for implementation**

Strategy	*Method*	*Evidence*	*Conclusions*
Passive dissemination	Mailing guidelines	Can influence awareness and knowledge of guidelines	Not sufficient to change practice
	Publishing in journals		
	Presenting findings at conferences	Innovative, user-friendly formats can help (Nuffield Institute for Health, 1994)	
Educational	Courses, conferences, workshops, professional meetings, educational materials	Ninety-nine studies of doctors showed doctors' behaviour can be modified and to some extent patient outcome improved, but effects are small (Davis *et al.*, 1995)	Educational interventions work best when they have an individualised 'active learning' component. Short courses, conferences and printed materials have little impact
Marketing	Out-reach visits (trained individuals visit practitioners in their own setting and talk one-to-one)	Eighteen studies showed a positive outcome and a few studies showed mixed effects on practice (Oxman *et al.*, 1995)	Effective because they are individualised and interactive
	Opinion leaders (targeting those with peer influence)		Needs more research and needs to clarify what opinion leaders actually do
Mass media	Mass media campaigns to disseminate evidence-based information, e.g. guidelines to public and practitioners	Have been effective in influencing the use of services (Grilli, 1999)	Potentially useful
Performance management	Audit and feedback – giving information to the practitioner about performance, usually with peer group comparisons	Review of 37 studies showed some impact on performance but only slight (Oxman *et al.*, 1995)	Can sometimes be effective in influencing practice but should not be relied upon alone
Incentives	Target payments	Review not yet available	

Passive dissemination strategies are probably the most commonly used for communicating the results of research. Publishing findings in a journal is one example. The Buckinghamshire guidelines had already been mailed to all GPs with a covering letter recommending their adoption – this is another example. This approach reflects a traditional industrial model – the Research, Development and Diffusion Model (Guba and Clark, 1966) – a rational sequence of events from basic to applied research, from development to packaging and then through a planned mass dissemination to a target audience. The assumption here is that the target audience will act as willing recipients of information and will make a rational decision to act on it, as long as it is good enough. At first sight, presenting findings at conferences or other educational events is also a passive dissemination strategy. Practitioners might have signed up for the event or decided to purchase the journal and read the article but the step to actually applying the findings in practice is a large one (see Chapter 9).

Sometimes educational events form part of a deliberate *educational strategy*. These work best when they draw on adult learning theory (Kolb, 1984) and seek actively to engage the learner, taking account of their own particular motivation. Small participative workshops are usually more successful at getting new ideas into practice than large conferences.

> ... the most beneficial are the ones [study days] where the morning is structured, possibly with lecture type sessions, and in the afternoon workshops, so that you get a chance to discuss and exchange ideas.
>
> (Midwife quoted in Meah *et al.*, 1996, p. 78)

It is also helpful if these educational strategies can link into the practitioner's own plans and priorities for continuing professional development.

Marketing strategies are borrowed from industry, particularly the pharmaceutical industry, and draw predominantly on two types of model:

- one concerned with the social influences on change – these focus on an understanding of the target audience in their own setting and of their social and professional networks and on the ways in which ideas are transmitted from one person to another

- diffusion of innovations models – concerned with measuring the process of adoption of (usually) concrete innovations such as new drugs or products through several stages, for example 'awareness, interest, trial and adoption' (Rogers, 1983). Rogers grouped adopters of innovation into five broad types:
  - the innovators
  - the early adopters
  - the early majority
  - the late majority
  - the laggards.

Identifying these can help in planning a strategy, taking account of probable sources of support and resistance.

The concept of *local opinion leaders* draws on both types of model:

> I think we all, or at least I have, at some time identified someone who I really respect, whose practice I would try.
>
> (Midwife quoted in Meah *et al.*, pp. 80–81)

While there is a lack of clear evidence about the effectiveness of opinion leaders, they are generally regarded as useful. In some areas this is being formalised by the appointment of 'link practitioners'.

Marketing approaches, particularly the use of out-reach visits, borrowed from the pharmaceutical industry seem to have an important role. The FACTs (Framework for Appropriate Care Throughout Sheffield) team have borrowed the techniques of pharmaceutical company representatives to try to persuade GPs in Sheffield to change their practice:

> The academic world prides itself on the sophistication of its theoretical understanding – impenetrability is almost a virtue. By contrast, the marketing world prides itself on the ease with which ideas can be grasped and the client's needs met. We believe that marketing techniques have much to offer in the attempt to translate research findings into action.
>
> (Eve *et al.*, 1997, p. 24)

However, this approach may well be off-putting for some practitioners.

Performance management and incentives strategies rest on very different assumptions. They are based on fairly simple models of human motivation – the rational–economic model, which asserts that we are motivated primarily by financial gain, and social models, which stress group conformity to peer pressures.

The overriding message from all the literature on strategies and methods for dissemination and implementation is that there are 'no magic bullets' (Oxman, 1995) and no single strategy will assure success. Instead, in most cases, a combination of methods, tailored to the specific circumstances, will be required. A further point to note is that all this research on strategies has been done on doctors. How far can the implications be extended to other groups of practitioners in health and social care? The complex issue of the generalisability of research findings is discussed further in Chapter 9.

Box 6: D&C in Buckinghamshire – Part 4

The Buckinghamshire GRiP team read the literature on implementation and tried to incorporate the central messages into their strategy. They used one particular GP, who was a member of the group but also a key opinion leader amongst his colleagues, in several ways. He spoke about the project at every opportunity at meetings of GPs and practice staff and made a series of informal out-reach visits to practices. The team booked sessions within existing continuing education courses, presented the work widely at conferences and other events, and produced articles for newspapers and professional journals.

---

3   And the user?

The attention so far has focused on dissemination to and implementation by practitioners. However, it is not only practitioners who need to know about the latest evidence of the effectiveness of treatments and services. Service-users need this information in order to make their own choices based on the research evidence and a whole range of other complex factors, some of which will be unique to them. In some situations it may be pressure from a well-informed patient that helps to change the practice of the health professional. In any case, the availability of clearly presented evidence-based information can help to change the patient–practitioner relationship from one in which the patient assumes the 'passive role of recipient of advice' to a 'partnership of shared decision-making [in which] the evidence about the effectiveness of treatments and their alternatives is made equally accessible to patients and professionals and is discussed openly and on equal terms, including the gaps in knowledge and areas of uncertainty' (Needham and Oliver, 1998, p. 87).

It may not be easy in practice for users to access this kind of information. However, self-help groups and consumer health information services have been influential in helping both groups and individuals obtain and make use of relevant research evidence. The Centre for Health Information Quality was set up with NHS Executive funding in 1997 to promote the development and use of high-quality evidence-based information for service-users (see the Appendix).

This was a major strand of the Buckinghamshire GRiP project. The team wanted to develop information for local women suffering from heavy periods so that they would know what treatment choices to expect. Rather than merely 'repackaging' the guidelines into non-technical language, the team wanted to identify the questions that women with this condition would want addressed. Informal discussions were held with small groups of women who had the condition. Had a leaflet been written as a simplified version of the guidelines (a common approach at that time), it would have focused on the technicalities of available treatments. As it was, two major issues emerged from the group discussions.

1 Women felt (or were made to feel) they were not justified in 'bothering the doctor' with this particular problem. Many who had sought help were told they 'just have to put up with it'. In many cases, the quality of their lives was drastically affected – some could not work or leave their home during their periods.

2 None of the women, including those who had been treated (many had D&C), had been informed at any stage that there was actually a choice of treatments (medical and surgical) available to them. All would have liked to have been given user-friendly information.

The pair of leaflets developed were designed to empower women to seek help and gave a framework for their consultation with the GP or nurse. All the treatment choices were described, based on the latest evidence of effectiveness and emphasising choice and personal preference. The leaflets were disseminated widely across the county and publicised through the local media and a workshop.

4   Successes and failures

What was the value of the Buckinghamshire GRiP project?

Members of the GRiP team are often asked whether the project was 'successful'. There were attempts to evaluate the work, both externally (Dopson and Gabbay, no date) and internally (Weinberg, 1993), but these were both 'after the event' and suffered from the project team's lack of clarity at the start of the project about what would constitute 'success'. This is perhaps inevitable in 'development' projects, which are deliberately exploratory and unstructured.

The original objective of reducing inappropriate D&Cs has undoubtedly been achieved – numbers have fallen dramatically. However, the figures had already fallen by 1993/4 (the proportion of all D&Cs done for menorrhagia fell from 67% to 49%) when the dissemination of the guidelines had hardly begun. Would the practice have changed anyway? It is almost impossible to judge. The project was well publicised locally and nationally and may have helped to bring down the numbers throughout the UK. On the other hand, there were many other sources carrying the same message.

If the project was directly responsible for reducing D&Cs in Buckinghamshire and, perhaps, improving the care offered to women with the condition, which elements of the 'multifaceted' strategy really made a difference? Was it the guidelines or the out-reach visits or the courses and conferences? Perhaps the information leaflets empowered local women to demand more appropriate care and treatment. There is, of course, no way of knowing.

The Buckinghamshire project was one of a set of demonstration projects christened GRiP (Getting Research into Practice) and later altered to GRiPP (and Purchasing) in the (then) Oxford Health Region. Four health authorities were asked to select specific topics where there was good evidence that local practice needed to change and to then do experimental work to try to make the change happen. The idea was to share the lessons with others on a national basis. Although each project developed its own methodology and approach to suit local circumstances, the sequence of activity was surprisingly consistent across the four projects. Some common lessons were identified and were 'branded' as the GRiP 'steps' (see Box 7 overleaf).

Box 7: The GRiP 'steps'

- *Choose* a topic which has local relevance and where existing practice is beginning to be questioned.

- *Involve* all the right people early in the project.

- *Find and appraise* all the relevant evidence (preferably involving the whole group to give them ownership of the evidence).

- *Carry out* a baseline audit of current practice.

- *Develop* local guidelines.

- *Use* a multifaceted strategy to implement the guidelines.

- *Develop* and disseminate information for service-users.

- *Plan* from the outset how to evaluate the impact of the work.

(Source: adapted from Needham, 1994)

These demonstration projects served a potentially useful purpose in describing a process which could be replicated by others with similar requirements. Many other regional GRiP-type projects have followed throughout the UK. The national Promoting Action on Clinical Effectiveness (PACE) programme (Dunning *et al.*, 1998), funded by the Department of Health, has built on the experience of GRiP. Another purpose has been to draw attention to important, if predictable, advice about communication, ownership and project management – messages which would, however, apply equally to any change management exercise.

A weakness of these projects is that they are all reviewed from the perspective of the project teams. This means they cannot throw light on the experience of those who have been targeted by the implementation strategies or explore any significant impact (or lack of it) on the practitioner's world.

How successful are national initiatives?

Alongside local efforts such as these there is a much larger-scale national effort to promote evidence-based practice. Two of the most important tools of this NHS-wide strategy are the *Effective Health Care Bulletins* and the *Cochrane Library*.

Effective Health Care Bulletins are distributed widely and freely in the NHS. They are systematic reviews produced in an accessible format with the implications for practice clearly presented. A survey by Walshe and Ham (1997) of all trusts and health authorities asked about their responses to three of the bulletins.

Many respondents were unable to say whether or not the Effective Health Care Bulletins' recommendations had been heeded. On two bulletins, four out of five H[ealth] A[uthoritie]s did not know what action, if any, their local trusts had taken ... Only 12 per cent said they had changed practice in response to the controversial recommendations of the bulletin on prostate surgery ...

(Walshe and Ham, 1997, p. 25)

These disappointing results throw the value of such strategies into question. Interestingly, the authors note that the bulletin which seemingly had the most impact (*Management of Cataracts*) was probably the one whose recommendations were most likely to reinforce current clinical thinking.

The *Cochrane Library*, with its regularly updated database of systematic reviews, is the key source of evidence about effectiveness. In the early days of its development, the database featured only studies of pregnancy and childbirth. Considerable efforts were made to disseminate it on disk to all obstetric units and health care libraries with the request that it should be made available to all practitioners and service-users to support policy and clinical decision making and informed choice.

The 32 midwives interviewed by Meah *et al.* in 1996 were all aware of the database and its value and some reported its use by their medical colleagues. None, however, had used it themselves. The reasons they gave were particularly revealing: it was available in the medical library which they were not allowed to use; or it was considered too expensive to buy – the cost of the database was under £100.

There are, without a doubt, various explanations for the failures described. One contributory factor may be a continued tendency to see the process of implementation as essentially 'a one-way "trickle-down" from research to the real world' (Eve *et al.*, 1997, p. 7) with the individual practitioner in a position to receive information and then make rational decisions about adoption. Eve continues:

In fact, the situation is more complicated than this. Practitioners managing the real world are often aware of their lack of knowledge and look to the research world for answers. Given that most of their energy is directed towards coping with today's problems, new knowledge tends to be utilised in a haphazard and intermittent way.

(Eve *et al.*, 1977, p. 7)

Many practitioners would, in any case, reject this role altogether. In a survey of 1226 professional grade social care staff by the Centre for Evidence-Based Social Services (Sheldon *et al.*, 1999), the respondents reported that the responsibility to keep up to date with research is both a departmental and a personal/professional responsibility. However, they saw the department as significantly more responsible than themselves. The Centre for Evidence-Based Social Services, of which Sheldon is Director, is seeking to change this attitude through an educational programme that aims to 'enable participants to evaluate research evidence and recognise the importance of using sound research evidence within the decision making process' (Spittlehouse, 1999).

Where practitioners are highly motivated to adopt an evidence-based approach, their good intentions are frequently frustrated by a complex web of restrictions, including lack of resources, time pressures, lack of access to information, lack of managerial vision and restrictive hierarchies. The midwives who opened this chapter gave this example:

> ... we've [clinical midwives] just done a thing [literature review] about cord care, and how to change it. We got together all the stuff, and it was obvious it [current practice] should be changed, and an infection control person [medic] came along with two pieces of research which were not particularly valid, but because they were his, that's it. We've left it now, nothing's going to be done. ...

> You can prove things until you are blue in the face, but at the end of the day, if the consultants don't want to do it, it won't be done.
>
> (Midwives quoted in Meah *et al.*, 1996, p. 80)

Movements for change

The strategies discussed in this chapter are all deliberate attempts to influence practitioners. However, change in health and social care practice has always been influenced by what are best regarded as social movements; not so much deliberate co-ordinated strategies for change as shifts in thinking whose origins and dynamics are difficult to pin down. Perhaps the best example is the sea change from the 1950s onwards favouring community care over residential care. To say this was an 'evidence-based change' in any straightforward way is difficult. Rather, it was the change in thinking that led practitioners and politicians to look for and value evidence demonstrating the adverse effects of institutions on individuals, and the favourable effects of alternatives to institutional care.

Such movements are very complex phenomena, influencing practitioners, service-user groups and others in a wide range of different fields. They do include deliberate, planned strategies to influence practice, of all the kinds referred to above, but the important point here is that movements like these both shape the agenda for change, prioritising evidence about some matters more than others, and shape the ideas of the people the strategy is trying to influence.

These remarks are equally true of the movement for 'evidence-based' practice in its current form, which prioritises the dissemination of evidence about effective, value-for-money interventions, and particularly the kind of evidence produced through experimental approaches. This movement has some support among some practitioners but, equally, others are antipathetic to it because they themselves prioritise other aspects of health and social care practice. Understandably, audiences will be much more receptive where the messages they receive correspond with what they think already than where the messages seem to support principles and policies with which they disagree.

Conclusion

Practitioners are increasingly being called upon to account for their own practice and required to identify, appraise and implement evidence relevant to their work. The policy frameworks in both health and social care (including 'best value' and 'clinical governance') are demanding new levels of co-ordinated policy (locally and nationally) to support and promote this approach. Policy directives and the developing work on strategies for change need to incorporate a greater understanding of the context in which the practitioner is working. On the other hand, the practitioner needs to scrutinise research findings in the light of a detailed knowledge of local circumstances and the practice of their own organisation. These issues are explored in the following chapters.

References

Antman, E. M., Lau, J., Kupelnick, B., Mosteller, F. and Chalmers, T. C. (1992) 'A comparison of results of meta-analyses of randomized control trials and recommendations of clinical experts', *Journal of the American Medical Association*, Vol. 268, No. 2, pp. 240–8.

Cheetham, J. (1994) 'The Social Work Research Centre at the University of Stirling: a profile', *Research on Social Work Practice*, Vol. 4, No. 1, pp. 89–100.

Cochrane, A. L. (1931/71, 1979) 'Critical review, with particular reference to the medical profession', in *Medicine for the Year 2000*, London, Office of Health Economics.

Coulter, A., Klassen, A., MacKenzie, I. Z. and McPherson, K. (1993) 'Diagnostic dilatation and curettage: is it used appropriately?', *British Medical Journal*, Vol. 306, pp. 236–9.

Davis, D. A., Thomson, M. A., Oxman, A. D. and Haynes, R. B. (1995) 'Changing physician performance: a systematic review of the effect of continuing medical education strategies', *Journal of the American Medical Association*, Vol. 274, No. 9, pp. 700–5.

Dopson, S. and Gabbay, J. (n.d.) 'Evaluation of the GRiPP Projects', unpublished internal report.

Dunning, M., Abi-Aad, G., Gilbert, D., Gillam, S. and Livett, H. (1998) *Turning Evidence into Everyday Practice*, London, King's Fund.

Eve, R., Golton, I., Hodgkin, P., Munro, J. and Musson, G. (1997) *Learning from FACTS: Lessons from the Framework for Appropriate Care Throughout Sheffield (FACTS) Project*, ScHARR Occasional Paper 97/3, University of Sheffield, School of Health and Related Research (ScHARR)

Grilli, R., Freemantle, N., Minozzi, S., Domenighetti, G. and Finer, D. (1999) 'Mass media interventions: effects on health services utilisation' (Cochrane Review), *The Cochrane Library*, Issue 4, Oxford: Update Software.

Guba, E. G. and Clark, D. L. (1966) *Effecting Change in Institutions of Higher Education*, Bloomington, Indiana, National Institute for the Study of Educational Change.

Hicks, C. and Hennessy, D. (1997) 'Mixed messages in nursing research: their contribution to the persisting hiatus between evidence and practice', *Journal of Advanced Nursing*, Vol. 25, pp. 595–601.

Hicks, C., Hennessy, D., Cooper, J. and Barwell, F. (1996) 'Investigating attitudes to research in primary health care teams', *Journal of Advanced Nursing*, Vol. 24, pp. 1033–41.

Holton, S. and Needham, G. (1995) *Successful Purchasing: From Information to Action*, London, King's Fund College.

Independent Review Group (1994) *A Wider Strategy for Research and Development Relating to Personal Social Services*, Report to the Director of Research and Development, Department of Health, by an independent review group (chaired by Gilbert Smith), London, The Stationery Office.

Knipschild, P. (1995) 'Some examples of systematic reviews', in Chalmers, I. and Altman, D. (eds) *Systematic Reviews*, London, British Medical Journal Publishing.

Kolb, D. A. (1984) *Experiential Learning: Experience as the Source of Learning and Development*, Englewood Cliffs, New Jersey, Prentice Hall.

Luker, K. A. and Kenrick, M. (1995) 'Towards knowledge-based practice: an evaluation of a method of dissemination', *International Journal of Nursing Studies*, Vol. 32, No. 1, pp. 59–67.

MacDonald, G. (1996) 'Evaluating the effectiveness of social interventions', in Oakley, A. and Roberts, H. (eds) *Evaluating Social Interventions*, pp. 39–62, Essex, Barnados.

Mann, T. (1996) *Clinical Guidelines: Using Clinical Guidelines to Improve Patient Care within the NHS*, London, Department of Health, NHS Executive.

Meah, S., Luker, K. A. and Cullum, N. A. (1996) 'An exploration of midwives' attitudes to research and perceived barriers to research utilisation', *Midwifery*, Vol. 12, pp. 73–84.

Munro, E. (1998) 'Improving social workers' knowledge base in child protection work', *British Journal of Social Work*, Vol. 28, pp. 89–105.

Needham, G. (1994) 'A GRiPPing yarn – getting research into practice: a case study', *Health Libraries Review*, Vol. 11, pp. 269–77.

Needham, G. and Oliver, S. (1998) 'Involving service users', in Bury, T. and Mead, J. (eds) *Evidence-based Healthcare: A Practical Guide for Therapists*, pp. 85–104, Oxford, Butterworth-Heinemann.

NHS Executive (1998) *Information for Health: An Information Strategy for the Modern NHS 1998–2005*, London, NHSE.

Nuffield Institute for Health, University of Leeds, Centre for Health Economics and NHS Centre for Reviews and Dissemination, University of York and Research Unit, Royal College of Physicians (1994) 'Implementing clinical practice guidelines', *Effective Health Care*, Vol. 8, pp. 1–12.

Oxman, A., Thomson, M. A., Davis, D. A. and Haynes, R. B. (1995) 'No magic bullets: a systematic review of 102 trials of interventions to improve professional practice', *Canadian Medical Association Journal*, Vol. 153, No. 10, pp. 1423–31.

Rogers, E. M. (1983) *Diffusion of Innovations*, London, Free Press.

Sheldon, B. *et al.* (1999) *Prospects for Evidence-Based Social Care: An Empirical Study*, Centre for Evidence-Based Social Services, University of Exeter.

Smith, L. N. (1994) 'An analysis and reflections on the quality of nursing research in 1992', *Journal of Advanced Nursing*, Vol. 19, pp. 385–93.

Spittlehouse, C. (1999) *CASP for Social Services; Final Project Report*, Oxford, CASP.

University of Leeds School of Public Health (1992) 'The treatment of persistent glue ear in children', *Effective Health Care*, Vol. 4, November.

Walshe, K. and Ham, C. (1997) 'Who's acting on the evidence?', *Health Services Journal*, 3 April, pp. 22–25.

Weinberg, J. (1993) 'Evaluation of the Process of the Buckinghamshire GRiPP Project', unpublished survey of stakeholders.

Chapter 8
Agency information for better practice

Roger Gomm

Introduction

Amina wants to enthuse her colleagues with some new ideas she has just picked up at a conference. As she drafts the script for a presentation to the staff meeting, she begins to think of the sort of questions colleagues or managers might ask her:

- How do our results compare with those described at the conference?
- What do we actually do, and how does this differ from what they do?
- Were they dealing with the same kinds of clients as we do?
- How many staff, of what kinds, working how many hours did they use? How does this compare with the number and kinds of staff we have and the way we deploy them?
- What was their non-staff budget, and how does it compare with ours?

There are two sides to these questions. The presenters at the conference may or may not have given Amina all the information she needed about *their* practice context. (This is considered further in Chapters 9 and 10.) But there is also Amina's side. Does she have access to the information needed to answer these questions? Her agency may actually be more successful for its clients, or more cost-effective in its operation, than the 'leading edge' practices she has just learned about. Alternatively, perhaps what enthused her would simply be impossible to emulate under her working circumstances. As Chapter 7 indicates, proposals for change are often met with resistance. But if there is no good evidence in favour of change, resisting it may be the more sensible policy. Answers to the kinds of questions above are the kinds of evidence that allow proposals for changing practice to be evaluated properly.

It is too much to expect any practitioner to carry all this information in her head. The important issue is whether Amina's agency is organised so that answers to these questions are easily and quickly available to people like her, at the time when she needs the information. In Chapter 7 there is a case study of different rates of D&C operations in various hospitals in Buckinghamshire. Box 1 in that chapter gives an example of the way in which routine record keeping can highlight important issues in service provision.

Agency records should provide evidence that:

- indicates what an agency is achieving currently, for whom, at what cost, and so on
- provides the basis for making decisions about agency development
- enables comparisons to be made with other similar agencies (such bench-marking should help practitioners to estimate whether more successful practice elsewhere would be possible for them)
- enables practitioners to compare their own performance with what has been shown through research or in demonstration projects
- allows practitioners to monitor the effects of changing practice, whether in the light of research findings or from local inspiration. For example, following clinical guidelines (Chapter 7, Section 2) implies monitoring the effect of doing so.

To make an informed choice about implementing the findings of research done elsewhere, practitioners need to know a great deal about their own practice first. The best place to find such information, in a form that is directly relevant to the practitioner's working circumstances, should be in the information routinely recorded in practice. But whether the answer will be found there depends largely on the quality of the agency's information management system.

1   Information for decision making

Decision support systems

The information practitioners need is the kind that helps them, and clients, to make decisions. Some decisions will be made at an individual or a case level centred mainly on service to a particular client. Information systems of this kind are often called 'decision support systems', but they would be more accurately called something like 'case decision support systems'. Client case notes or patient records are nearly always the core information in such systems.

Other decisions might be made about matters such as: how a practitioner should deploy her time between different tasks, or the eligibility criteria for service, or the opening hours of the office; how to decide between alternative expenditures or whether to be more proactive in attracting clients of particular types, for example, from minority ethnic backgrounds. Information systems supporting decisions of this more strategic kind are often called 'management decision support information systems' or 'management information systems' for short. The same system may well serve both purposes. Indeed, data aggregated from the individual records of many clients usually lies at the core of a management information system in health and social care. (See Table 1.)

Table 1   **Information for making case and strategic decisions**

Type of information	(Case) decision support system	Management decision support system
1 Information about clients	Service-relevant information for each client: e.g. age, gender, ethnicity, diagnosis, mode of access, date of access to service; preferences for particular kinds of treatment Recorded complaints	Numbers of clients falling into each service-relevant category Data on client satisfaction/ dissatisfaction Geographical distribution of clients Analysis of complaints
2 Information about procedures	What has been done for each particular client? – the client's service record or case notes. Who did it? What it is planned to do in the future for each particular client: e.g. care plans	What has been done for clients falling into particular categories, e.g. men compared with women, older people compared with younger? High dependency compared with lower dependency? Which staff/kinds of staff achieve most with which kinds of client?
3 Information about resources/costs	What resources were used in providing a service to this particular client? (This may entail a question about a client's eligibility to receive a particular *level* of service)	How are resources deployed to different categories of client? What resources were used that cannot be attributed to any client: e.g. overheads, rent, heating, lighting, recruitment and training costs?
4 Measures and records	What data are collected, when and how? Are the data most relevant for making decisions about and with individuals?	What data are collected, when and how? Are the data most relevant for making strategic decisions?
5 Information about outcomes (since the idea of an 'outcome' assumes change, information about outcomes needs information about the client before an intervention – baseline information)	What has been achieved for this client (so far)? Putting 3 and 5 together, how much did it cost to achieve these outcomes?	What has been achieved for all clients and for clients falling into particular categories? Putting 3 and 5 together, what is the cost per outcome?
6 Information about aspirations	What were the aims, objectives, targets for this client? Putting 5 and 6 together, how far have they been achieved? Putting 3, 4 and 5 together, were the outcomes for this client achieved within budget targets, or did resource shortages prevent the targets being met?	What are the targets for all clients? And for clients of particular kinds? Putting 5 and 6 together, how far were they achieved? Putting 3, 5 and 6 together, were the outcomes for all clients achieved within budget targets or did resource shortages prevent the targets being met?

This chapter is largely about information for making 'management' decisions, which will affect several clients rather than any one in particular. But the 'manager' here may be just a practitioner trying to manage her own practice better.

There are times when the only way to answer the questions in the third column of Table 1 is through specially designed, one-off evaluation research projects. Perhaps an unbiased independent judgement is required, or perhaps a special effort has to be made to track clients after they have lost contact with the agency. But specially mounted evaluation studies are expensive. Sometimes the fact that they have to be commissioned at all results from shortcomings in the way an agency documents its own activities. If there were an adequate system of information management, evaluation might become a routine process of interpreting the records and discussing the results with staff and service-users.

Increasingly, the people who commission or otherwise fund services require monitoring systems so that evaluation is a routine and ongoing feature of a service. Similarly, the many performance indicators imposed on the NHS (Merry, 1997) and social services or social work departments (Audit Commission, 1995a, 1998; LGMB, 1997) require the routine collection of data to establish whether performance targets have been met. Action research (see Chapter 5) also relies on establishing sound monitoring systems to ensure that lessons can be learned from the research.

It is not easy to design good information management systems (Sheaff, 1995). The task requires a great deal of foresight about what questions the system should be answering. For example, if there is no provision to record the ethnic affiliation of clients, the system will not be able to answer questions bearing on equal opportunities issues. Or if there is no provision for recording the start and finish time of contacts with clients, the system will not be able to give a picture of how much time is spent with clients, or with clients of particular types, or how much time they spend waiting around for delayed appointments.

Modelling what happens: a caution referral scheme

Designing information management systems also requires the identification of all, or at least most, of the common sequences of action in an agency. This does not mean that each act in each sequence has to be recorded, far from it. But unless there is an accurate model of what usually happens in the agency, it will be impossible to make a sensible decision about what to record and how to record it. Figure 1 (overleaf) is a simple example from a drugs caution referral scheme, which is then discussed further.

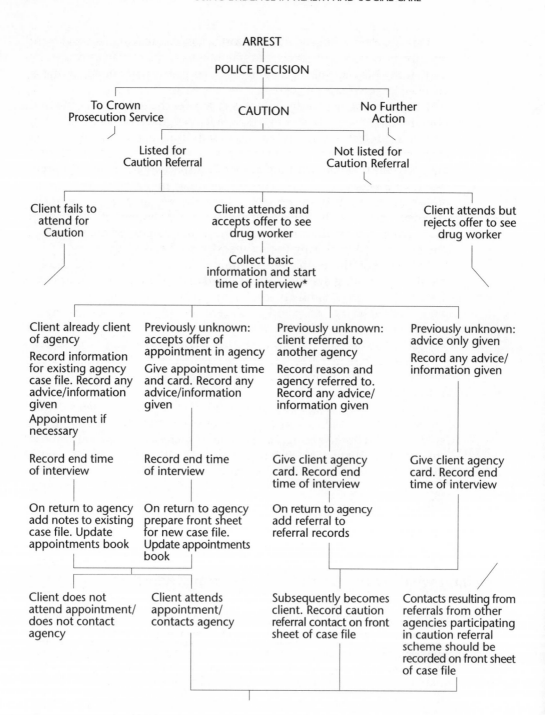

* Client's name and address should not be recorded on the caution referral day sheet

Figure 1   **Activity pathways and data flows in a drugs caution referral scheme**

Imagine that Amina works in a street drugs agency which has been asked to participate in a caution referral scheme on a six-month pilot basis (see Figure 1), along with other agencies offering advice and information about alcoholism, debt, homelessness, and so on. What enthused Amina was a glowing report of the success of a drugs caution referral scheme elsewhere. But many reports of success are exaggerated and the fact that something is successful in one place is no guarantee that it will be successful in another. So what Amina's agency needs to know is whether using its resources in this way will be a good investment for them. The resources are six hours a fortnight spent giving drugs-related information at the police station to offenders who are attending to be formally cautioned for an offence; that is 72 staff hours in six months that might be spent otherwise. In addition, funding might become available for this service at a later date, and the agency wants to gather the kind of evidence that would support a funding bid if this proves to be a worthwhile activity. For both purposes there needs to be a monitoring system that will answer the following basic questions.

• How much time in the police station was actually spent in contact with clients?

• How many offenders, over a time period, elect to see a drugs worker?

Of these:

• How many were given advice and of what kinds?

• How many subsequently became clients of the agency?

Of these:

• What happened to them as clients of the agency?

Figure 2 (overleaf) shows the form used to capture the relevant data. Note how it reflects the activity pathways and data flows in Figure 1.

At the end of the six-month period, Amina's agency was able to produce an analysis, part of which is shown in Table 2 (overleaf).

Much of the time spent at the police station was not spent in contact with clients. Although not shown in Table 2, the data collected showed that most of the clients who elected to see a drugs worker were cautioned for minor offences such as possessing small amounts of cannabis. These are the kinds of people who usually do not consider themselves to have a 'drug problem' and are not usually dealt with by a drugs agency. The 'time conversion rate' showed that it took 76 hours' attendance at the police station to generate three new clients for the agency and to provide some kind of advice or information to 32 clients in all: the latter at a cost to the agency of around £1000 or £31 per head.

Whether this is 'costly' or not depends on how productively the agency could have used that time in other ways. Making that judgement depends on knowing how time is actually spent on other agency activities, and to what effect (see Chapter 10). As always, decisions are likely to involve considerations that escape the recording system. Here, for example, the

CAUTION REFERRAL DAY SHEET:	WORKER:	DATE:
Staff arrival time	Staff departure time	
Number of clients listed for referral		
Number of clients who did not attend		
Number of clients who opted not to see drug worker		
Number of clients already clients of the agency		
Number of clients seen by drug worker		

CLIENT No. 1	Start time:	Finish time:	Total contact time:
Gender	Kind of advice given (specify)		
Age	Referral to other agency (state agency)		
Ethnic group	Appointment made and case file opened		
Main drug of use	Other notes		
Offence			
Already agency client Y/N			

CLIENT No. 2	Start time:	Finish time:	Total contact time:
Gender	Kind of advice given (specify)		

Figure 2   **Form used to capture data for a drugs caution referral scheme**

benefit of earning the goodwill of the police by participating is set against the possible cost of becoming too closely identified with the criminal justice system for the liking of some of the agency's clients.

2   Information technology and information management

The discussion so far applies to information in any medium, whether it is stored in the practitioner's or the manager's head, on paper or electronically. As noted in Chapter 7, the *Information for Health* strategy has been an important component of the attempt to promote evidence-based

Table 2 **Part of the synopsis of six months' experience of a drugs caution referral scheme**

Number of clients listed by police for drugs referral	47
Number of listed clients who attended for caution	35
Number of attending clients seen by drugs worker	32
Time spent in contact with clients (hours)	21
Time spent at police station not in contact with clients (hours)	55
Total hours spent at police station (x)	76
Number of clients given advice/information only	18
Number of clients referred to another agency	2
Number who were existing clients of the agency	5
Number of clients for whom drug agency appointment was made (new clients only)	7
Number of clients who kept appointment at drugs agency (y)	3
Time conversion rate: hours required to recruit one new agency client (x/y)	25

practice in the NHS. This recognises that practitioners' knowledge about their own practice is as important as their knowledge about research findings. It includes an investment programme for information technology for both purposes (NHS Executive, 1998). Modern information technology offers two possibilities that are difficult to achieve in paper-based systems (Glastonbury, 1995): integrated management information systems and automation.

Integrated management information systems

With paper-based systems there are strict limits to the number of purposes a single system can serve and agencies usually operate with multiple systems of information management. Then the same information often has to be entered into several systems. Considerable effort may be needed to bring together the information from one system and merge it with that from another. Sometimes there can be long delays before all parts of the system are up to date with each other. Service-users often complain that they have to supply the same information repeatedly as they pass from practitioner to practitioner. Modern electronic information technology allows for single entries of data to serve many purposes, single updating entries to update the whole system, and each item of information to be brought to bear on the others. Once the NHS has established a UK-wide electronic patient-record system, it should be possible for A&E staff immediately to access and update a patient's full medical record, as long as they know the patient's name and one other unique identifying characteristic. The estimated date of installation of this system is 2007 (Fieldbaum and Dick, 1997).

Automation

In medicine, input can be automated by collecting data directly from diagnostic or therapeutic equipment, or with bar-code readers. But for most systems automated analysis is the greatest benefit. For example, if the recording for the drugs caution referral system was paper-based, all the analysis shown in Table 2 had to be done by someone reading 12 day sheets (Figure 2) plus the case records of the seven clients who were given appointments, and transferring the information into another format. Had the data been input directly into a relational database, only a few key strokes or mouse clicks would be necessary to make the computer read all the forms and to print out a 'report' with the information required, in text, tabular or graphic format. With an automated information system it is easy to display matters such as gender, age or ethnic differences among the clients, cross-tabulated with the kind of offence committed. Some of the more sophisticated information management systems used in acute medicine can use the same database to create reports of different kinds for different readers – for example, using 'MCI' (myocardial infarction) for medical readers and 'heart attack' for patients or carers – and some systems offer a choice of different languages (NHS Training Directorate, 1996). (Geographical information systems are covered in Chapter 11, Section 2.)

Information technology has made the greatest inroads into acute medical care (Audit Commission, 1995b), as exemplified below.

The Glasgow Nephrology Information System

This system (described by Simpson and Gordon, 1998) links the in-patient nephrology unit at the Glasgow Royal Infirmary and seven out-patient clinics with the biochemistry, haematology, microbiology and tissue-typing laboratories, the pharmacy, hospital social work, dieticians and the ambulance service. It can be consulted by everyone involved in patient care, including nursing staff, PAMs, secretaries, and medical records and ambulance staff. Confidentiality is handled by passwords and by classifying some information as off-limits to some users. An automatic audit trail records who has consulted the system, what they have viewed and what, if any, data they have input. There are 50 terminals including mobile terminals for use on ward rounds. In 1998 the system was handling data on 10,500 patients. It has the capacity to handle data on millions.

The centre-piece of the system is the database of individual patient records. These include the clinical history and the current clinical management plan, updated by the doctor during consultations, usually with patient and doctor viewing the screen display together and deciding what entries should be made. The system allows the doctor to access clinical guidelines, diagnostic algorithms and other decision-making aids, which can be used by merging them with the data on the particular patient. Prescriptions can be written on screen and transmitted directly to the pharmacy, but they also give the pharmacist an opportunity to comment and perhaps to suggest a modification, which will appear in the client's electronic file for the doctor's consideration. Diagnostic tests can be ordered similarly and the results transmitted directly to the patient's file, alerting the relevant doctor that this new information has arrived. Nominated nurses and PAMs can 'eavesdrop' on all this and input the detailed care plans for their own speciality.

Data such as those from biochemistry tests before and after haemato-dialysis are automatically fed to the patient's file, and compared with pre-set targets. If the results are above or below a specified level the system prints out a warning alerting staff to the need for action.

The system will also do the following.

- Display the appointments record of each patient.
- List staff who play key roles for each patient.
- Prepare and transmit labels for samples, laboratory request forms and prescriptions.
- Order transport.
- Automatically record the patient's progress through the system as data are entered.
- Automatically record whether the patient's appointment started on time and how long it lasted.
- Generate letters to the patient's GP, by automatically addressing them and merging patient data with a letter written by the hospital doctor.
- Generate recall letters to non-attenders, and letters to GPs about persistent non-attenders.
- Generate a discharge report and reports to social services.
- Keep an up-to-date record of bed-state.
- Automatically issue prompts to appropriate staff concerning matters such as outstanding tests, or other actions that are needed.
- Prepare an overarching list of missing information for the unit administrator.
- Prepare reports for clinical audit purposes: electronic links with the Scottish Renal Register allow local performance to be compared with performance elsewhere.
- Prepare reports on compliance with advice from bodies such as the Committee on Safety of Medicines.
- Access research databases such as the Cochrane Collaboration's databases (see Chapter 7, Sections 2 and 4).
- Automatically record activities such as lengths of time spent in dialysis, and expenditures such as the costs of medication and clinical tests.
- Debit the unit's account for the cost of medication and tests.
- Issue prompts and action plans following, for example, a worrying change in blood chemistry, or the death of a patient.

To expand the final point on the list: simply recording a patient's death generates an action plan telling staff that a death certificate, printed by the computer, will need to be completed and signed; that a report will be needed for the Procurator Fiscal (it would be the Coroner in England, Wales or Northern Ireland); that appointments will have to be arranged with relatives, and so on. These prompts remain outstanding until they are cancelled by recording that the tasks have been completed. Recording the death will generate a request for a necropsy; cancel outstanding out-patient appointments, transport arrangements and prescriptions; alter the ward's bed-state status report; update the unit's morbidity and mortality records; and list the death for consideration at the next weekly review.

If Amina had been working in an agency with an information system like this then it would probably provide her with all the information she required to answer the questions posed at the beginning of this chapter.

Different agencies, different information problems

The Glasgow Nephrology System, in 1998, gives a glimpse of what information management will probably look like in many, if not most, medical specialities by 2020. But some areas of health and social care lend themselves more easily than others to the design of integrated systems like this. Although it manages a large amount of information, the Glasgow system still has to deal with only a limited range of types of information, because there is only a limited number of ways in which kidneys fail and only a limited range of procedures for treating such conditions. Designing an integrated and generic system for a primary health care team would be much more challenging (Mackintosh and Shakespeare, 1995). Again, in nephrology many of the crucial data for decision making are quantitative: for example, the results of urine testing or haematolysis readings. This allows the system to be pre-set to alert staff immediately to worryingly high or low readings, but merely to store for later consideration those within acceptable limits. It is difficult to think of much information from the sphere of social work, for example, that could be managed in this way (Glastonbury, 1995).

Table 3 identifies some further differences between agencies. It suggests it is easier to design an information system for assembly-line elective surgery, where the same few kinds of operation are done repeatedly at much the same cost each time, and where the follow-up of patients is possible. It would be more difficult to do this for general practice where patients present with a multiplicity of conditions of different severity and where following them all up is not feasible. Agencies such as street drugs agencies have particular problems in collecting the kind of information that allows them to judge longer-term outcomes, because their clients so often disappear without trace (Edmunds et al., 1998). Practitioners in

Table 3 Factors making it easier or harder to design an integrated information management system

Factor	Design easier, e.g. in an acute medical speciality	Design harder, e.g. in a street drugs agency
1 Information about clients	Clients are willing to provide or have no choice about providing information about themselves Contact can be maintained with clients for periods long enough to evaluate what the agency has achieved for them, or the clients can be tracked over a longer period	Clients may be unwilling to disclose information about themselves and sometimes provide misleading information. Asking for 'too much' information may undermine trust Clients often lose contact with the agency so there is no way of knowing what has been achieved for many of them in the longer term
2 Categorisation	There are well-established systems for classifying clients, conditions, activities, etc. with a well-known vocabulary; for example, the nosological categories of the Reid codes or ICD10 in medicine (Walker, 1995; Campbell and Payne, 1994) and standardised clinical procedures with common names	The field of practice does not have any standardised system of classification, or it is subject to multiple and incompatible systems of classification; for example, mixtures from medicine, social work and/or the criminal justice system
3 Information about procedures	The work of the agency consists of well-defined sets of activities of relatively few kinds which have recognisable starting and finishing points Staff are 'specialists'; space and equipment are dedicated to particular purposes	The work of the agency is 'client-led' and directed towards resolving or ameliorating a wide variety of problems. It is difficult to specify the purpose of each episode of client contact and therefore difficult to say whether this has been successful Staff are generalists
4 Information about resource deployment	Because of factors 1–3 it is relatively easy to cost the different activities of the agency, in terms of time and money, and to cost the service provided for each client or kind of client	Because of factors 1–3 it is more difficult to cost the different activities of the agency in terms of time or money
5 Information about outcomes	The agency is dedicated to achieving a few well-defined outcomes (see 2 and 3) which: are easy to recognise if they are achieved; are achieved while the clients are in contact with the agency (see 1); can be costed in terms of the procedures used to achieve them (see 4)	Desirable and feasible outcomes are multiple and difficult to specify. Clients often lose contact with the agency before any evaluation of the agency's work with them can be made. It is difficult to cost the benefits of particular procedures carried out with and for clients
6 Confidentiality	The system for managing the information is contained within a single confidentiality system; for example, the NHS	Exchanging information about clients between agencies is often frustrated because of confidentiality considerations
7 Dependence on other agencies	Outcomes for clients are largely attributable to the activities of the agencies within the same integrated management information system and do not depend on the performance of other agencies	Outcomes for clients are often crucially dependent on the performance of agencies with different information systems (for example, the Community Drug and Alcohol Team, the police, the probation service, the housing department, social services). What happens to clients is often difficult to attribute to agency actions
8 Freedom to design own information system	The agency can choose what information to collect and in what format, or the information it has to collect to satisfy funders, auditors, etc. is consistent with its own information requirements	The agency has to collect and report information in ways determined by those who commission and regulate its services. This includes data which are not useful for its own purposes
9 Resources for managing information	There is adequate time, resources and equipment to collect and manage the information needed	There are only limited resources of time and capital for collecting and managing the information needed

health promotion may have no difficulties in recording what information they provide for whom and at what cost, but they may be unable to collect any data on their effectiveness at all, if the effects they are trying to achieve are long-term changes in health-related behaviour (Tudor-Smith *et al.*, 1998).

However, what is an 'outcome' is largely a matter of definition. All agencies can measure some outcomes. In the example of the drugs caution referral scheme it was impossible for the agency to collect comprehensive information about long-term outcomes such as offenders ceasing to use drugs or not reoffending. However, it was possible to collect information about numbers of offenders taking up the offer to see a drugs worker, numbers who received advice about the needle and syringe exchange, numbers who kept an appointment at the agency, numbers who came back again, and so on. All these are outcomes of a drugs worker attending the police station during cautioning. Recording data about them produces some useful lessons.

Another issue is the question of whose requirements for information the system should be designed to serve. A system precisely designed to provide the information requested by clients might be very different from one precisely designed to provide the information most wanted by practitioners or by managers, by an inspection team or by financial auditors, by the politicians of a local authority or by a government ministry. Considerations of cost almost always set limits on the number of different requirements an information system can serve. The important cost is the labour cost of collecting, inputting, processing and reporting. Whatever kind of system is used, there will be a point at which the cost of increasing the range of data collected will be greater than the benefits of having the additional information (Sheaff, 1995). Costs such as this may be shown in fewer clients being served, in data being collected but rarely used, or in decisions being delayed until someone can find the time to look at the records. Over and above initial investment costs, the point at which collecting additional data becomes more costly than useful is reached much more quickly with paper-based or non-automated electronic systems. But even the most powerful integrated and automated electronic system is unlikely to be able to handle *all* the data wanted by *everyone* without diverting resources from some other activity that is more worth while – according to someone at least. A good recording system provides the right information to the right people at the right time. But who are the right people and what is the right information can be contestable matters.

3   Joined-up recording in research and practice

Few health and social care organisations make full use of all the information they routinely collect. Many still rely on paper-based records which take an inordinate amount of time to analyse. However, underuse may also be a problem of the human organisation of practice. Using agency information requires a timetable of events for producing reports, considering them and making decisions about them.

Practice reviews

The Glasgow Nephrology Information System described in Section 2 automatically produces a report on about 150 patients for a weekly team meeting, highlighting patients approaching dialysis, and showing details of biochemistry, diet, fistulae, suitability for home dialysis, potential for transplantation, operation scheduling and other data needed for decisions and a smooth change to a life on dialysis.

> Preparing the report takes two minutes; previously, it took a secretary four to six hours. ... Patients with specific problems are 'flagged'. The flag or marker can be set at any terminal by any staff member, and stays 'on' until it is dealt with at the meeting. Operation waiting lists, patient transfers, and deaths are also reviewed. Morbidity, mortality, and other statistical analyses are available.
>
> (Simpson and Gordon, 1998, p. 1656)

This is not just a case review meeting. As the reference to 'morbidity, mortality and other statistical analyses' indicates, it is also part of the clinical audit system; a regular peer review of the evidence generated from practice, comparing this, where possible, with evidence from other sources (Kogan *et al.*, 1995).

Processes such as clinical audit, practice evaluation or quality assurance ask the questions 'How are we doing?' and 'How could we do better?' A great deal can be learned by a team comparing its own performance this year with last year's, or comparing the outcomes of one kind of intervention with those from another. But simply making in-house comparisons does not tell a team whether they are performing as well as others are performing elsewhere, or as well as they possibly could. In helping to answer the question 'How are we doing?', research evidence can provide appropriate standards of comparison. And in helping to answer the question 'How could we do better?', research evidence can be used to help a team select between treatments on the basis of which of them research shows to be the most effective and/or cost-effective.

> Although the purpose of audit is to evaluate how closely our own practice is to best practice, research aims to establish what that best practice actually is. So, if research tells you that 70 per cent of depressed

patients are significantly improved by a particular combination of imipramine and cognitive-behavioural therapy, then your audit might indicate that your own depressed patients, given that treatment, are improving at that rate.

The data you collect should be able to tell you why you are exceeding that standard of practice or not meeting it. For example, by measuring people's depression at admission, using the same inventory as the original outcome research, you should be able to see if your patients are more severely depressed than theirs were, or if they had longer or shorter time for therapy, and so on.

(Firth-Cozens, 1993, p. 9)

Matters are not usually quite as straightforward as Jenny Firth-Cozens describes. There is rarely just one single authoritative piece of research to consider. More often there are several with findings that are not always compatible with each other. Systematic reviews or meta-analyses are not always available (see Chapter 7, Sections 2 and 4) and sometimes there is no relevant research at all. And there are formidable problems in applying the findings of research done in one place to the circumstances of practice in another – as is discussed further in Chapters 9 and 10.

However, Firth-Cozens does capture the important way in which research findings can inform practice reviews and lead to more effective practice. This entails squaring-up data on local practice so that point-by-point comparisons can be made with what was found in research, as in the second paragraph of the quotation above. That, in turn, means making decisions to do this in advance. In Firth-Cozen's example, the questionnaire measuring degrees of depression, as used in the research study, would have to be administered before implementing treatments, not afterwards.

Standardisation or diversity?

It is difficult, if not impossible, to compare the performance of different agencies if they all do something different and record information in different ways. The same is true if different researchers use incommensurate systems of measuring and define terms in radically different ways.

The 'obvious' solution to this problem is standardisation both of agency record keeping *and* of research practice. There has been considerable pressure in this direction in health and social care. In the example from Glasgow (Section 2), bench-marking the renal unit's performance on the data from the Scottish Renal Registry means using a similar methodology of measurement and recording to that used in the Registry. The format used in the Cochrane database (Chapter 7, Sections 2 and 4) has tended to become a standard for researchers engaged in clinical effectiveness research. This has influenced the choice of recording systems in medical practice, so that practice outcomes can be compared with research findings and vice versa. Similar reasons explain national projects to produce standardised outcome measures for social work in child care (Ward and Jackson, 1991; Davies, 1998) and the programme for evidence-based probation practice (Home Office, 1999). The use of performance indicators (McColl *et al.*, 1998), inspection standards (in residential care) or local-authority-wide systems for abuse management, or of standardised 'returns' of data to central government departments, again all have standardising implications for practice, recording and research.

The 'obvious' solution, however, gives rise to some equally obvious problems.

- Standardising on one model of best practice may prevent agencies achieving something else which is 'best practice' according to another standard of judgement. For example, researchers in the disabilities field have been highly critical of the hidden assumptions about disabled people built into commonly used outcome measures (Zeibland *et al.*, 1993; Priestley, 1995). Criticism about the misleading nature of performance indicator data has been widespread (for example, Hamblin, 1998).

- Different information-users have different information requirements. Integrated information systems designed to serve a wide range of information needs may be unwieldy. Compromises may produce a system that suits no one. It has proved difficult to persuade GPs to provide consultants with the information the consultants want and vice versa (McKenna *et al.*, 1994) and the gap between health and social care is even greater.

- Deciding what to record and how to record it always means deciding what not to record and how not to record it. Thus standardisation in recording runs the risk of no one noticing something that may turn out to be extremely important. There is always a danger of 'check-list' decision making, based on the data recorded, ignoring other factors which are relevant but do not feature in the database.

- Progress in research depends to some extent on the creativity of researchers in finding new questions to ask. Standardising research questions and procedures tends to inhibit this, even if standardisation does lead to the accumulation of knowledge that will 'fit together'.

The relative merits of standardisation versus diversity are not easy to decide. On the one hand, there is the argument that the areas of pure and applied science that have made most progress are those which make the most use of standard classification systems and vocabularies. For example, without standardisation of nosology in medicine it is impossible for medical researchers to communicate with each other effectively, or to communicate with doctors. By contrast, in areas such as psychotherapy or social work, there is such a bewildering variety of vocabularies that it is sometimes difficult to know whether two exponents are talking about the same conditions, outcomes or interventions, or about something completely different (Macdonald, 1999). On the other hand, there is the argument that standardisation is always standardisation on someone's terms and usually tends to embed and perpetuate the ideas of the powerful.

However, if research is to influence practice, and vice versa, there has to be some sharing of a common language in which researchers report their findings and practitioners record their practice.

Conclusion

The main message of this chapter is that unless practitioners know what they themselves are achieving and how they are doing it, evidence from research will only be of limited use to them. If they do not know this, much of all that effort put into disseminating research evidence (discussed in Chapter 7) will be wasted. As noted in Chapter 7, one of the problems of applying research findings in practice is that researchers and practitioners often do not 'speak the same language'. However, this chapter noted that, increasingly, the way agencies make records is influenced by the format of research findings, while the targets set by national government for service agencies have also set the research agenda. For example, the declaration of targets for the *Health of the Nation* strategy in England, its counterparts in other parts of the UK and their successors immediately stimulated research around the target issues. Agency recording systems are increasingly becoming the lingua franca between researchers and practitioners.

This is the first of three chapters with the common theme that, in order to apply research in practice, practitioners have to compare and contrast the circumstances of their own practice with the circumstances under which the relevant research was conducted. This chapter dealt with one side of this: the practice context. The next two chapters deal with the other side.

References

Audit Commission (1995a) *Local Authority Performance Indicators*, Vols 1 and 2 and *Appendix to Volumes 1 and 2*, London, Audit Commission.

Audit Commission (1995b) *For Your Information: A Study of Information Management Systems in the Acute Hospital*, London, HMSO.

Audit Commission (1998) *Consultation on the Local Government Performance Indicators*, London, Audit Commission.

Campbell, J. and Payne, T. (1994) 'A comparison of four schemes for coding of problem lists', *Proceedings of the American Symposium on Computer Applications for Medical Care 1994*, pp. 201–5.

Davies, C. (1998) 'Developing interests in childcare outcome measurement: a central government perspective', *Children and Society*, Vol. 12, pp. 155–60.

Edmunds, M., May, T., Hearnden, I. and Hough, M. (1998) *Arrest Referral: Emerging Lessons from Research*, Paper 23, London, Central Drugs Prevention Unit, Home Office.

Fieldbaum, E. and Dick, R. (1997) *Electronic Patient Records, Smart Cards and Confidentiality*, London, Financial Times Pharmaceutical and Healthcare Publishing.

Firth-Cozens, J. (1993) *Audit in Mental Health Services*, Hove, Lawrence Erlbaum Associates.

Glastonbury, B. (1995) *Computers in Social Work*, Basingstoke, Macmillan.

Hamblin, R. (1998) 'The wrong target', *Health Service Journal*, 2 April, pp. 28–31.

Home Office (1999) *Evidence Based Practice in the Probation Service*, London, Home Office.

Kogan, M., Redfern, S., Kober, A., Norman, I., Packwood, T. and Robinson, S. (1995) *Making Use of Clinical Audit*, Buckingham, Open University Press.

Local Government Management Board (LGMB) (1997) *Performance Indicators*, London, LGMB.

Macdonald, G. (1999) 'Social work and its evaluation: a methodological dilemma?', in Williams, F., Popay, J. and Oakley, A. (eds) *Welfare Research: A Critical Review*, London, UCL Press.

Mackintosh, C. and Shakespeare, G. (1995) 'Primary health care and general practice', in Sheaff, R. and Peel, V. (eds) *Managing Health Service Information Systems: An Introduction*, pp. 47–64, Buckingham, Open University Press.

McColl, A., Roderick, P., Gabbay, J., Smith, H. and Moore, M. (1998) 'Performance indicators for primary care groups: an evidence-based approach', *British Medical Journal*, Vol. 317, pp. 1354–60.

McKenna, M., Paxton, R. and Grant, W. (1994) 'Communications between a multiagency mental health service and general practitioners: are standardisation and audit possible?', *Journal of Mental Health*, Vol. 3, No. 4, pp. 513–20.

Merry, P. (1997) *1996–97 NHS Handbook*, London, NAHAT/JMH Publishing.

National Health Service Executive (1998) *Information for Health: An Information Strategy for the Modern NHS 1998–2005*, Leeds, NHS Executive.

National Health Service Training Directorate (1996) *Just for the Record: A Guide to Record Keeping for Health Care Professionals*, Bristol, NHS Training Directorate.

Priestley, M. (1995) 'Dropping 'E's': the missing link in quality assurance for disabled people', *Critical Social Policy*, Autumn 44/45, pp. 7–21.

Sheaff, R. (1995) 'Informatics and health care', in Sheaff, R. and Peel, V. (eds) *Managing Health Service Information Systems: An Introduction*, pp. 1–11, Buckingham, Open University Press.

Sheaff, R. and Peel, V. (eds) *Managing Health Service Information Systems: An Introduction*, Buckingham, Open University Press.

Simpson, K. and Gordon, M. (1998) 'The anatomy of a clinical information system', *British Medical Journal*, Vol. 316, 30 May, pp. 1655–58.

Tudor-Smith, C., Nutbeam, D., Moore, L. and Catford, J. (1998) 'Effects of the Heartbeat Wales programme over five years on behavioural risks for cardiovascular disease: quasi-experimental comparison of results from Wales and a matched reference area', *British Medical Journal*, Vol. 316, pp. 818–22.

Walker, H. (1995) 'Classification and coding', in Sheaff, R. and Peel, V. (eds) *Managing Health Service Information Systems: An Introduction*, pp. 133–41, Buckingham, Open University Press.

Ward, H. and Jackson, S. (1991) 'Developing outcome measures in child care', *British Journal of Social Work*, Vol. 21, pp. 393–99.

Zeibland, S., Fitzpatrick, R. and Jenkinson, C. (1993) 'Tacit models of disability underlying health status instruments', *Social Science and Medicine*, Vol. 37, pp. 69–75.

Chapter 9
Would it work here?

Roger Gomm

Introduction

This chapter is about transferring research findings to somewhere else where they might be implemented. Usually there are differences in client characteristics, staff expertise and commitment, institutional structures and levels of resourcing. Paul Nutting and Larry Green, writing as practitioners in primary health care, draw attention to the different orientations of researchers and practitioners:

> First, biomedical research isolates single diseases or disease processes. Much of the research enterprise is designed to understand further the biomolecular mechanisms, diagnoses, and treatments of specific diseases. This often requires that the disease is studied in its fully developed form and in patients without other diseases that would confound the study. In many cases it requires as the focus of study a specific organ, tissue, cell, or intracellular process. Second, disease is studied in highly selected patients. In order to focus on a specific disease mechanism or treatment effect, most medical research carefully restricts the characteristics of the patients under study. Often studies emphasize male adults in their middle years with fully developed disease, without other co-morbidity, and in whom adherence to the protocol can be carefully controlled. Third, most medical research is designed to evaluate single interventions. Although many clinical trials compare special interventions, they are rarely combined in a single arm of the trial in the ways that they are actually used in primary care. Fourth, biomedical research tends to prefer 'hard' outcomes, such as death or changes in physical measurements. Less attention is devoted to key personal consequences of effective primary care such as relief of suffering, a sense of having been understood, and the preservation and restoration of function. Finally, the strong focus on disease mechanisms often purposefully excludes the effects of the patients' physical and psychosocial environments, the powerful effects of the physician–patient relationship, and the multiple effects of the system factors inherent in the organization and financing of primary health care services – all of which are central to the environment of primary care.
>
> (Nutting and Green, 1994, pp. 156–8)

The main burden of the quotation is that the circumstances of experimental research may bear little relationship to what usually happens in practice. It is important not to assume that this difficulty is especially associated with experimental research. It is very likely that a piece of research done in the ordinary, workaday circumstances of a particular residential home for older people will not apply directly to another residential home, because its ordinary, workaday circumstances will be different in significant respects. The results of qualitative research, which might have a bearing on 'physician–patient relationships' and 'a sense of being understood', are even more difficult to transfer from one place to another.

There are two aspects of applying research in practice. The first is making the decision about whether some research finding is worth the attempt to put it into practice and estimating the feasibility of doing so. The second is about the logistics of actually doing this. The latter is the process of implementing change in practice. There is no great difference here between implementing and bedding down changes that have been inspired by research findings, and implementing those that are foisted on an agency by an external funder, or those that arise from the enthusiasms of staff.

Many of the difficulties of implementing research in practice discussed in Chapter 7 are first and foremost difficulties of change management (Keep, 1998). Action research was dealt with in Chapter 5 and change management and action research can be very similar. This current chapter then is about the first aspect of application. It is about answering the question 'Would it work here?'

1   The context dependence of outcomes

The outcomes of most procedures in health and social care are context-dependent. A large number of factors will determine what happens. These are likely to appear in different constellations, both for different clients and between different practice locations. Figure 1 gives a very simple picture of the kinds of factors that might vary from agency to agency. While each agency might be applying a procedure that looks the same, variations in other kinds of factor are likely to produce different outcomes.

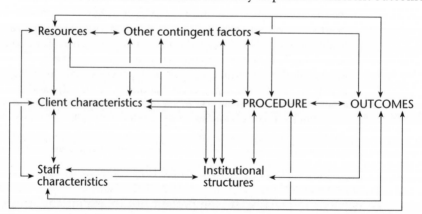

Figure 1   **The context dependence of outcomes**

Figure 1 can be fleshed out with the quotation from Nutting and Green by comparing the location of some randomised trial of a clinical procedure with a situation in everyday practice, as in Table 1 (overleaf). In principle the table would apply to any situation where research of any kind was done in a different situation from that in the place where an attempt is being made to apply its findings.

Table 1 has only one column for the practice setting. In reality there should be a different column for each different general practice. Each will represent a different constellation of variables. Even if a piece of experimental research is replicated – copied in exactly the same way – it is still likely to produce different results. That is the point of meta-analyses (see Chapter 7). And when something like the same procedures are implemented in *different* everyday practice settings, diversity of outcome is just what is to be expected. The results of experimental research are just as 'context-dependent' as the results from everyday practice. The difference is that experimental researchers rig the context as far as possible to reduce the number of variables at play to avoid 'confounding' (see Chapter 3). But what are confounding variables for the experimental researcher are the very stuff of everyday practice.

2 Specified procedures

Unless research produces something like a recipe, a set of instructions, guidelines or a protocol, it is virtually impossible for a practitioner to know what to do in order to do 'the same' in an attempt to produce similar outcomes. Some kinds of research are more transferable for this reason than others.

The example in Table 1 was of a procedure that is among the most easy to specify and standardise – administering a drug. Pharmaceuticals are manufactured to high quality control standards; each pill is identical. Protocols for administering drugs can be written unambiguously and followed with ease. Other practice procedures may be much more difficult to specify.

> It is now clear from meta-analyses of almost 500 evaluative studies (e.g. Smith, Glass and Miller, 1980) that most forms of psychotherapy and counselling are approximately 50 per cent more likely to produce an improvement than would occur without treatment, provided the outcome is assessed from the client's subjective reports. These same meta-analyses mostly fail to show any difference between different forms of treatment, no matter how different in philosophy ... or how different the procedures ... and no matter what the disorder being treated. ... The non-specificity of treatment is confirmed by the failure to demonstrate any effect of training on the effectiveness of therapy (e.g. the meta-analysis of Berman and Norton, 1985). One is driven to the simple conclusion that psychotherapists do not know what they are doing and cannot train others to do it, whatever it is.
>
> (Howarth, 1989, p. 150, cited in Spinelli, 1994, pp. 76–77)

Table 1 **Differences between the context of research and the context of practice**

	The context of the research study, for example a pharmaceutical trial	The context in everyday practice, for example general practice
Client characteristics	The subjects are hand-picked to eliminate confounding variables. For example, they fall within a narrow age span, they are suffering from only one condition, their diagnosis is certain. Their understanding of participation is that they are involved in a research study but they do not know whether they are receiving the drug or a placebo, or which of two active treatments they are receiving	The patients choose themselves for presentation. They are of diverse ages, they are often suffering from several medical conditions, their diagnosis may be uncertain. Their understanding of the situation is that they are ill and want the doctor to make them better. They assume that whatever the doctor does is an attempt to make them better
Resources	Funded by a drugs company, the trial is well resourced, with dedicated time to conduct it. Cost considerations do not enter into the decisions to treat, and research considerations inhibit expending more resources on any subject other than those the research protocol dictates	The treatment of these patients, as for all others, has to be accomplished with limited resources of time and budgets. Practitioners may attempt to expend more resources on those in greatest need, and it is most unlikely that each patient is treated in the same standardised way
Practitioner characteristics	Staff have been specially inducted in how to administer the drug and are monitored to make sure they do no more and no less than the protocol dictates	The practitioner may be unfamiliar with the drug. His or her concerns will be fitting the treatment to the patient, and not following a standardised set of procedures
Institutional structures	The study was done in a hospital where drugs were administered by staff	The practitioner works in general practice. Patients are required to administer their own medication at home
Other contingencies	The research is designed as far as possible to eliminate chance occurrences	All kinds of things happen in practice: a locum changes the medication for one client; a patient cannot get her prescription dispensed; and so on
Measures	Baseline and outcome measures may have been designed precisely for the purpose of the trial and the trial will have been organised to facilitate the necessary measurement	The measures used in the trial may not be the same as those used in the practice. It may be difficult to measure in the same way as in the trial. It may not be possible to know whether the practice is achieving better or worse results than the trial (see Chapter 8)
Procedures	The procedures for administering the drug are tightly specified as part of the research design	The procedures adopted are custom-built for each patient. Patient choice plays some part in the process
Outcomes	Because of the research design, outcomes can be attributed to the effect of the drug as administered according to the research protocol	Because of the many factors that vary from patient to patient, it will be unclear how outcomes were produced

The important issue here is the non-specificity of treatment. It is rarely clear whether two practitioners doing 'counselling' or 'psychotherapy' are doing the same thing. Therapists attempt to make their practice client-specific, so it is not at all clear that a counsellor counselling one client is using the same procedure as the same counsellor counselling another. Studies which demonstrate that counselling can produce high levels of client satisfaction also seem to demonstrate that the critical factors are the personal characteristics of the counsellor (Howe, 1993), rather than the procedures she uses (see also Berman and Norton, 1985). In terms of Figure 1 then, 'counselling' and 'psychotherapy' seem to produce outcomes which are more dependent on the characteristics of practitioners than on the procedures adopted or the theory behind them.

By contrast, the research literature gives a clearer picture of the effectiveness of cognitive behavioural therapies (Drury *et al.*, 1996a and b; Kemp *et al.*, 1996). It can do so because in cognitive behavioural therapy the procedures are much more clearly specified and more standardised in application, and the practice is aimed at achieving a few simple, measurable outcomes. For the 'talking treatments' there is then the puzzle of deciding whether cognitive behavioural therapy is really more effective than counselling, or whether the former simply lends itself better to evaluation than the latter (Stiles, 1994; Sechrest, 1994).

But the important point here is that research on the effectiveness of cognitive behavioural therapies can tell others what to do in order to produce the same effects, while, seemingly, research on the effectiveness of psychotherapy and counselling cannot.

There are often no fixed meanings for terms used widely in practice. This gives rise to many opportunities for practitioners to believe that they are doing the same as something being done elsewhere, when actually they are doing something different. For example, within a single county council area, Gomm (1996, p. 3) found 12 different patterns of what practitioners called 'care management' in mental health and 10 arrangements called 'community mental health teams', giving rise to the possibility of 120 different combinations. He also found practitioners using the term 'key worker' in at least 15 different ways. Similarly, much of the research on the effectiveness of care (or case) management in mental health founders on researchers not specifying what they mean by the term (Brugha and Glover, 1998).

3 Mapping contexts

Figure 1 and Table 1 suggest that what works under some circumstances for some clients may not work for the same clients under other circumstances, or for different clients under the same circumstances. Thus judging the possibility of emulating what was reported in a research study entails answering the following questions.

- *Are the circumstances of our practice sufficiently similar to those of the research context to make it a good bet that what worked in the research will work for us?*

And:

- *In so far as there are differences, how feasible and how desirable would it be to change the context of our practice to bring it into line with that described in the research?*

Much the same headings as in Figure 1 and Table 1 can be used to represent the mapping exercise needed (Table 2 opposite).

Published research studies will rarely provide all the information needed about the research location. It may also be rather difficult for a team to answer all the questions for its own context and practice (see Chapter 8). But the better the answers to the questions in the first two columns of Table 2, the easier it will be to approach the more difficult questions in the last column.

To illustrate this kind of mapping, a case study of some action research will be used. Here the salient question is not 'Would it work here? but 'Why did it work in one place and not another?' These are slightly different questions, but the logic of answering them is essentially the same.

4 Why it worked in Kirkholt but not somewhere else

The Kirkholt Burglary Prevention Project in Rochdale (Forrester *et al.*, 1988, 1990; Pawson and Tilley, 1997, pp. 127–52) is regarded as an exemplar of good practice in crime prevention. Crime and fear of crime are major causes of ill health and disease and, hence, should be of interest to community health practitioners. They are major associates of the problems dealt with by social workers. Health visitors, district nurses, CPNs, social workers and housing workers may find themselves all involved together in activities related to crime prevention and victim support in inter-agency projects such as those under the Single Regeneration Budget Programme, Health Action Zone Projects, projects arising from the 1998 New Deal for Communities programme, and especially in the multi-agency crime and disorder strategies initiated by the Crime and Disorder Act 1998.

As social services and social work departments increasingly merge with housing departments, so more social workers are becoming involved in projects to regenerate the fabric and community life of decaying estates. These projects usually have a crime prevention objective among others. Crime and disorder is becoming everyone's business in health and social care. Moreover, all community projects, whatever they are focused on, can have secondary effects, such as improving people's sense of controlling their own lives, giving some of them valuable social roles to play and generally improving sociability in an area (Hunt, 1989).

Table 2   Cross-mapping the context of research and the context of practice

	The context of the research study	The practices and context of practice now	The desirability/feasibility of changing the practice procedures and context to match those of the research study
1 Client characteristics	What were the salient characteristics of their clients?	What are the salient characteristics of our clients?	Where there is a mismatch, could we and should we change our client mix?
2 Resources	What resources were used in producing the outcomes: staff time, money, equipment, space, and so on?	What resources do we expend for similar purposes for similar clients?	Have we got the resources to emulate practice in the research study? Would it be feasible/desirable to enhance or redeploy our resources?
3 Practitioner characteristics	What were the salient characteristics of the practitioners in terms of expertise, experience, commitment?	What are the salient characteristics of our practitioners?	In so far as there is a mismatch, would it be desirable/feasible to recruit different staff, invest in training, go through a team-building exercise, etc.?
4 Institutional structures	How far were the outcomes dependent on, for example, the departmental structure of the agencies featured in the research, or on co-operation with other agencies?	How far do institutional structures or inter-agency relationships determine our practice?	In so far as there are differences, would it be feasible/desirable to change the institutional framework in which we practise?
5 Measures	What baseline, outcome and other measures were used?	Do we use the same measures/could we use the same measures?	Would it be desirable to change the way in which we measure and record our practice?
6 Procedures	What exactly was done in the research study location which led to the outcomes reported?	Do we do exactly the same, or something different?	In so far as there are differences, would it be desirable/feasible to change what we do?
7 Outcomes	What were the outcomes, for whom (see 1) and what are they attributable to (see 2 to 6)? What was the cost per client (1 + 2)? What was the cost per procedure (2 + 6)? What was the cost per successful outcome (2 + 6 + 7)?	What are our outcomes of the same kind? Are they achieved for the same clients as in the research study? What do we achieve that was not achieved in the research study? To what are our outcomes attributable? What do we spend per client/procedure? What does it cost us to produce a successful outcome?	In so far as our outcomes are different, what are the differences attributable to (any of 1 to 6)? Are there outcomes we are not achieving/not achieving to the same degree which would be desirable/affordable for us to achieve? Could we achieve the same at a lower cost? Are we achieving some things now that we would have to forgo in order to emulate the practices in the research study?

Table 3   Outcomes of the Kirkholt anti-burglary project compared with one attempt to replicate it elsewhere

| Project | Number of burglaries per year | | | | Burglaries per 100 households |
	Year before project	After 1 year of project	After 2 years of project	After 3 years of project	Change over life of project
Kirkholt	526	233	167	132	Drop from 25% to 6% (3 years)
Safer Cities	571	694	991	N/A	Rise from 9% to 12.5% (2 years)

(Source: based on Pawson and Tilley, 1997, pp. 128–32)

Table 3 gives the outcome data for the Kirkholt project and for another project which was inspired by Kirkholt and implemented (later) under the aegis of the Safer Cities programme. There were several attempts to clone Kirkholt in the Safer Cities programme (Tilley, 1993, 1996) with variable degrees of success. Only one of them is featured here. Table 3 shows that the Kirkholt project was highly successful, but that the emulation was not. Kirkholt's reduction in burglaries was accomplished against a rise in surrounding areas, and nationally, while in the replica the rate of increase was almost the same as on surrounding estates.

So why was there a difference in outcome? Some purchase on this question can be gained by doing a cross-mapping exercise similar to that suggested in Table 2, but using some side headings more appropriate to these kinds of community project (see Table 4 opposite).

As Pawson and Tilley say (1997, p. 138), listing comparisons and contrasts like this can go on almost indefinitely as long as the information is available in sufficient detail to allow it. But it takes some inspiration, not to say guesswork, to identify the likely causes of success in one area and failure in another. At first glance, differences in the resourcing of the projects, in the size and nature of the communities, and in the characteristics of the local crime patterns seem likely to be crucial contextual differences to which differences in outcome could be attributed. But this is being wise after the event. It is worth trying to think of some questions the Safer City team should have asked about the Kirkholt project *before* they tried to emulate it. Here are some.

- *Based on Kirkholt what would be a reasonable number of households for the project to cover, given that we've only got £38,000 to spend over two and a half years?*

Kirkholt spent £82,917 over two and a half years (including some start-up costs): £36 per household. If, as it seems, some 855 burglaries were prevented in two and a half years, that is a cost of about £97 per burglary prevented. On this basis, the Safer Cities project was financed to deal with only about 1055 households adequately (not 8000), and it did not manage to reduce the burglary rate overall. This looks like a

Table 4 **Cross-mapping the characteristics of Kirkholt and the replication neighbourhood**

Characteristic	Kirkholt	Safer Cities
Resourcing	Very well resourced, at approximately £99,500 p.a., for 2280 households	Poorly resourced, at approximately £38,000 p.a., for 8000 households
Scale	2280 households	8000 households
Crime rate	Very high crime rate. Burglaries at 25% before project compared with national average of 5%	Moderate crime rate. Burglaries at 9% before project compared with national average of 5%
Main types of burglary	49% of burglaries involved electricity and gas meters	Few households with electricity and gas meters and few burglaries featured them
Community	Self-contained estate clearly bounded by roads. Outsiders easily identifiable. Culturally homogeneous: white working class. Initial suspicion and hostility to authority. Few obvious community leaders	No clear boundaries to the estate. No obvious limits to the community with much through pedestrian and car traffic. Culturally homogeneous: white working class. Less antipathy to authority, but few obvious community leaders
Organisation/ personnel	Multi-agency: Manchester University supplying the research expertise. Alternately led by the police and the probation service, with social services and housing department staff involved. Project offices adjacent to housing office on estate	Multi-agency, including academic support from University, but with police and probation as the main players. No clear overall leadership
Procedures	1 Improved ease of reporting crime and increased contacts with crime prevention services 2 Removal of coin-in-slot meters 3 Formation of mini Neighbourhood Watch schemes ('cocoons') eventually incorporating 90% of households 4 Target hardening. Security improved for all victims' homes. Victims introduced to cocoon members	1 Improved ease of reporting crime and increased contacts with crime prevention services 2 Formation of mini Neighbourhood Watch groups ('cocoons') but these only developed to include 25% of households 3 Target hardening for victims but only for council and housing association tenants

(Source: based on Pawson and Tilley, 1997, pp. 128–32)

familiar syndrome of trying to emulate a well-resourced demonstration project on the cheap, with the usual dismal results.

- *Given that Kirkholt featured a programme of crime surveillance by the community, were there any important characteristics of the community present in Kirkholt and absent in our proposed project area?*

Both areas looked unpromising for initiatives of the Neighbourhood Watch type but Kirkholt was an estate with clear territorial boundaries, such that strangers were easily identifiable; this is important if burglars were outsiders. It was a smallish estate where most people knew each other. Given its size, there was a possibility of creating blanket coverage by 'cocoons'. If burglars were mainly residents of the estate, the characteristics of the community would make it more likely that they would know about increased community surveillance and the increased risk of detection, about the removal of slot meters, the target hardening and the reduced risk of successful burglaries. The Safer Cities project area lacked many of these characteristics.

- *Does burglary have the same pattern in both areas and, hence, will measures adopted in Kirkholt work similarly in our area?*

In Kirkholt, burglary from slot meters predominated. Their removal from houses probably accounted for a very large percentage of the fall in burglaries. It is almost certainly the case that some of the 'burglaries' prevented were actually perpetrated by householders breaking into their own meters, and then reporting these as burglaries. In so far as much of Kirkholt's success was preventing thefts from slot meters, it was unlikely to be transferable to another area where such machines were rare.

Theorising is inevitable, and useful

Other equally enlightening questions might be asked. Some more will be said about 'target hardening' later but there is more than a simple cross-mapping of features between different areas going on here. What there is, in addition, is some theorising. This is nothing very grand but some commonsensical theories offered as possible explanations of how things hang together and why interventions have the effects they do.

So what is it about Kirkholt as a place that makes it possible to trigger what mechanism to produce these outcomes? Some of Pawson and Tilley's ideas are shown in Table 5 (opposite).

A similar kind of theorising was necessary to make sense of Tables 1 and 2. The results are shown in Table 6.

There are several things to be said about theorising in this way. First, it is highly speculative. It is wise not to become too attached to any such theory because it may be wrong. Second, it comes cheap. Most people can generate many theories linking context and mechanism to outcomes in a relatively short period of time. Third, this kind of theorising is inevitable. It is virtually impossible to not do it. Since it is inevitable, it is important to get it out in the open so that the ideas can be inspected to see whether they really are credible. As Howe has argued for social work, the problem in linking 'theory to practice' is that practitioners do it all the time, but rarely notice what theories they are actually using (Howe, 1987, p. 1). A fourth point is that explanatory ideas of this kind provide a good starting point for looking at the published literature. This frames the questions research is needed to answer, and does so in a way that will be closely related to practical concerns. Looking again at Table 5, it is easy to see how Pawson and Tilley's little bits of theory would guide them in searching the research literature for confirmation or disconfirmation.

Table 5 **Theorising the links between context, mechanism and outcomes in Kirkholt**

Context	+ Mechanism	= Outcome
Something about Kirkholt	+ *Something about the project*	= *Dramatically reduced rate of burglary*
A high crime rate area marked by very high rates of burglary	+ Security upgrading of previously burgled premises to increase difficulty and risk of apprehension in burgling particularly easy properties	= Lower rate of re-victimisation and a reduced burglary rate overall
High numbers of pre-payment meters, with a high proportion of burglaries involving cash from meters	+ Removal of cash meters reduces incentive to burgle (or fake burglaries) by decreasing actual or perceived rewards	= A reduction in percentage of burglaries involving meter theft; a reduced risk of burglary at dwellings from which meters are removed; and a reduced burglary rate overall
A medium-sized, socially homogeneous, clearly defined estate with little through-traffic. Easy transmission of 'news' from person to person	+ Cocoon home-watch increases perceived risks of recognition of offenders, knowledge among would-be offenders of decreasing rewards for break-ins, plus heightened levels of social control	= A reduced burglary rate overall and a general reduction in crime and incivilities

(Source: based on Pawson and Tilley, 1997, p. 134)

Table 6 **Comparing context, mechanism and outcome in a research study with context, mechanism and outcome in practice**

Context	+ Mechanism	= Outcome
Something about the research location	+ Some of the activities carried out there	= Produced the outcomes reported
Something about our practice context	+ Some of the procedures we follow	= Produces the pattern of our outcomes

So, a fifth point here is that the literature can be read in a rough-and-ready experimentalist way, posing hypotheses and seeing whether they are disconfirmed by published studies, along the lines of 'natural experiments' (see Chapter 3). For example:

> Is it true that burglary prevention projects are only successful in clearly defined, socially homogeneous neighbourhoods?

If so, there should be no examples of successful burglary reduction projects in other kinds of neighbourhood. Or, all other things being equal, burglary reduction projects should be successful in proportion to the extent that the areas have clear natural boundaries, and a fairly stable and socially homogeneous population. Or:

Is it usually true that the main mechanism for burglary reduction is a raised expectation of being apprehended?

If so, there should be no examples of successful projects which did not include some successful means for disseminating information about the increased risk of being caught.

In some areas, context–mechanism–outcome connections are well established by research. For example, much is known about the biochemical mechanisms through which drugs work or the physiological mechanisms through which wounds heal, and the circumstances (contexts) necessary for these mechanisms to operate. Similarly, there is an aspect of the Kirkholt project which is, indeed, well established by research.

Robust mechanisms

In the Kirkholt project and in the Safer Cities replica one set of crime prevention procedures is implicated that is reliable and robust and will transfer to a wide range of different neighbourhoods. This is so-called 'target hardening'. Research studies from many industrialised countries have demonstrated that, unless remedial action is taken, the risk of a residence being burgled increases with the number of times it is burgled. For someone who has been burgled once, their risk of being burgled again increases markedly; twice, and it increases even more (Farrell and Pease, 1993; Pawson and Tilley, 1997, pp. 135–42). Similar regularities are shown in many kinds of victimisation including graffiti, vandalism (Burquest et al., 1992), littering, child abuse, thefts of cars from particular streets or car parks, domestic violence and racial attacks (Sampson and Phillips, 1992). Previous offences predict further offences (Farrell et al., 1995). In other contexts this provides the rationale for police policies of 'zero tolerance' ('nip it in the bud quick'), and it is part of the reason why the police prefer to 'target' their activities, rather than adopt the publicly popular policy of putting more officers on regular beats, which is less effective in reducing crime. Regarding burglary, it has inspired the impressively effective policy of target hardening the residences of people who have been burgled and doing so as quickly as possible. Target hardening can include a wide range of techniques such as property marking, instant repairs after a break-in, better security against un-authorised access, burglar alarms, and direct or CCTV surveillance (Anderson et al., 1995).

'Cocooning' is not an inevitable part of target hardening but it was used in both projects. Neighbourhood Watch initiatives keep the whole neighbourhood under surveillance, but cocoons are small groups of neighbours who focus surveillance on people or properties at particular risk. The technique has also proved valuable in cases of domestic violence and it seems to work under a wide range of different circumstances: another robust mechanism.

Target hardening was involved in both projects. Looking at Table 3, it might seem sensible to say that the Safer Cities project had no effects. But that would be erroneous. True, it did not lower the overall burglary rate. But there are no interventions that have *no* effects. In fact, target hardening worked to reduce repeat victimisation in the Safer Cities project just as it did in the Kirkholt project. However, in the former only some of the targets were hardened. Burglars, seemingly, avoided the hardened targets and transferred their attention to other easy access property on the same estate. In the Safer Cities project *some people* were made less vulnerable to burglary. But, since the overall burglary rate did not fall, *some people* must have been made *more* vulnerable.

Among the many mechanisms at play in producing outcomes, some will only be triggered under rather peculiar circumstances, while others will operate much more generally. Perhaps the most valuable function that research plays for practice is in identifying robust mechanisms of the latter kind. But beware, the same mechanism that makes an opiate an effective painkiller also makes it an addictive drug. The context determines how the mechanism works. In the same way, the law of repeat victimisation was at work in Kirkholt and in the Safer Cities replica, but with different outcomes in the different contexts.

What works for whom under what circumstances?

This highlights an important set of problems in applying research to practice – the issue of 'What works for whom?' In research reports, outcomes are often expressed without differentiating outcomes for different people: often as average ('mean') or majority effects. The expression of outcomes in terms of a reduction in overall burglary rate is another example of this. A fall in the overall burglary rate in an area might mean that *everyone* became less vulnerable to burglary. It might also mean *some kinds of people* became *less vulnerable*, and *some other kinds of people* became *more vulnerable*, but that there were more of the former and fewer of the latter.

Health and social care interventions often carry a risk of disadvantaging some groups of people to the benefit of some others. The national initiative on hospital waiting lists in the 1990s is an example (Hamblin, 1998). The policy of 'prioritising the most severely mentally ill' in community mental health services is another (Department of Health, 1995). Drug testing in prisons has probably reduced the overall

Table 7   **The five outcome groups for any health and social care intervention**

For any intervention there will be				
1 People for whom the intervention has only benefits	2 People for whom the intervention produces benefits which outweigh the disadvantages	3 People for whom the intervention has very little or no effect at all	4 People for whom the intervention produces disadvantages which outweigh the advantages	5 People for whom the intervention has only disadvantages

consumption of drugs among prisoners but it has also shifted some users from easily detectable cannabis, to the more dangerous and less detectable heroin (Edgar and O'Donnell, 1998).

This can be expressed more formally as in Table 7.

All people being equal, practitioners would want to tailor their practice so that there were more people in categories 1 and 2 than in 4 and 5. But all people are not equal and they should not be treated equally in practice. In many situations practitioners will be quite willing for an intervention to create large numbers of minimally disadvantaged people, in order to produce large benefits for a few whose needs are regarded as taking moral priority: perhaps simply by doing nothing at all for the former, and much for the latter. There will be no attempt here to discuss the host of difficult ethical and political issues involved in making decisions about distributing the benefits and spreading the misery. For this chapter the important point is this. Unless a research study identifies the five outcome groups in Table 7 (or at least the three 1 + 2, 3, and 4 + 5), it will be difficult to predict the out-turns of applying the research findings to a particular practice population.

What makes this a particularly acute problem is that the mix of clients dealt with by any real-life practice will almost never match the mix of clients featured in a research study (Nutting and Green, 1994, pp. 156–8). In a study, perhaps 10% of the subjects experienced severe drug side-effects. In a GP's caseload there might be as few as none or as many as 50% or more vulnerable to this. Unless the study identifies contra-indications for prescribing the drug, the GP cannot apply the findings to maximise the number of beneficiaries and minimise the number of people harmed by the intervention.

Or again, perhaps a piece of evaluation research shows that an independent supported living scheme was successful for the majority of *their* clients. But does it distinguish between those kinds of clients for whom it is successful and those for whom it is not? Maybe another practice population contains a majority of the latter.

Thus, in appraising the transferability of published research, it is important to see whether the authors specify *differential* outcomes for particular client groups in such a way that would enable practitioners to identify these different groups in their own setting.

Institutional arrangements

To implement research usually means reconfiguring the context of practice so that it matches the context in which the research was done. This is relatively easy where the changes are within the discretion of a single practitioner or a small team. The easiest kind of research finding to implement is where a doctor simply substitutes one pharmaceutical product for another. However, much health and social care practice entails multidisciplinary, and often multi-agency, collaboration. Then setting up the conditions under which the research findings might be implemented successfully may require protracted negotiations between different disciplines or different agencies. The result may be a compromise between the interests of different stakeholder groups creating a situation very different from that needed to produce the same outcomes as in the original research. Perhaps something like this happened in the Safer Cities project. Its institutional arrangements, particularly those about the leadership of the project, were certainly different from those which obtained in Kirkholt (see Table 3).

In reading research with a view to judging its transferability with regard to institutional arrangements, there are four questions.

1 Are the outcomes of this intervention likely to be sensitive to institutional arrangements?
2 Does the research report clearly specify the institutional set-up?
3 Could we manage to negotiate similar institutional arrangements in our locale?
4 What might be the disadvantages of changing institutional arrangements? Would these outweigh any advantages?

For example, some research literature on multi-agency community mental health teams suggests that their success is crucially dependent on inter-agency agreements that insulate team members from managerial demands emanating from outside the team, which might otherwise pull team members in different directions (Ford et al., 1993).

Competing priorities

Another important question is whether trying to achieve some outcomes through applying research findings in practice might prevent the achievement of some other outcomes which are equally or more desirable. Much research is single-minded: stripped down to pursue the answers to just one or two questions. But, in practice, practitioners and agencies have to juggle many competing, and perhaps mutually incompatible, objectives. The success of the Kirkholt project may be derived from its close focus on preventing not just burglary but burglaries involving slot meters in particular, whereas the Safer Cities project diffused its effectiveness by trying to tackle crime on a broader front.

Whatever the truth of this, in attempting to implement research in practice, agencies often adopt more general objectives than in the original research, or they combine the objectives of the research with others with which they are incompatible. There is a very strong pressure to do this wherever there is a process of bidding for funding. Then agencies and partnerships often promise to do more than they could ever reasonably be expected to achieve, and they may promise to do this for less money than would make even some of it possible.

Again, where service-users are allowed a significant voice in determining practice, they may choose what the research shows is less effective. For example, police–public consultation usually shows a very strong demand for more police on the beat (Bucke, 1995). This might help reduce the fear of crime (Bennett, 1991). But reducing the fear of crime by beat policing and reducing the committing of crime by targeting particular locations and kinds of offences may be mutually incompatible objectives within a fixed budget.

Commitment and expertise

Success in achieving outcomes may be due, partially at least, to the staff involved in the research being better trained or better briefed than staff might be in routine practice. Or perhaps the staff or the service-users involved in research or a demonstration project were motivated and enthused by this (Sapsford and Abbott, 1992, p. 105; Bowling, 1997, p. 137). As Sheldon and his colleagues (1998) note, if the success of stroke units demonstrated through research is due mainly to the commitment of their staff, this is a very expensive way of securing commitment.

Enhanced commitment is particularly likely where the research originated from the bright ideas of staff or service-users, as in most 'action research' (see Chapter 5). One of the 'robust mechanisms' referred to earlier is that people are generally more committed if they dreamed up the scheme in the first place. On transferring research to practice elsewhere, this commitment and enthusiasm may be difficult to replicate. Indeed, in so far as a demand for change implies the deficiency of current practice, transferring from research to practice may often be associated with resentment and obstructionism (see Chapter 7).

It is always worth looking closely at published research to see what it says about the expertise and training of the practitioners involved, and about the ways in which they and service-users were briefed, consulted with, and so on. The key question is whether the same levels of expertise and commitment that were associated with successful outcomes in the research programme can be replicated in practice elsewhere. A formal 'training needs analysis' may be necessary to identify whether staff have the requisite expertise, and to commission training where they do not (Buckley and Caple, 1990; Wright, 1999). All but the most minor changes in practice require briefings, consultations and perhaps 'team-building' exercises. And successful team building requires that participants are given some significant ability to determine what the team will do, and how it will do it.

Conclusion

This latter point poses a dilemma. On the one hand, it seems that the most effective way of transferring research findings to practice is to reorganise practice so that it precisely matches the conditions under which the research was done. On the other hand, to transfer research findings into practice means: generating commitment among practitioners and service-users; satisfying their preferences (which may be different from those featured in the research); respecting their judgement and areas of discretion; combining the pursuit of outcomes featured in research with other equally desirable ones; and managing local obstacles which did not impact on the research, but cannot be eliminated from the practice setting. In these regards, transferring research into practice often means radically departing from what was done in the research programme or demonstration project. Doing the same thing differently with the same results is a difficult trick to pull off.

This chapter explained why this is a difficult trick. It is because of the context dependence of the outcomes of any health or social care intervention – whether routine or part of a research project. Some suggestions have been made for how to approach this set of difficulties. These involve:

- cross-mapping between a local practice setting and what is reported in the research project
- theorising what mechanisms were at play in producing outcomes for the research and how contexts, mechanisms and outcomes were related in the research
- estimating whether the same set of relationships can be reproduced in practice
- deciding whether it would be desirable to change practice in a way that would increase the chances of achieving results similar to or better than those shown in the research
- considering what disadvantageous effects might arise from changing practice more closely to match what happened in the research programme.

Published research will often be inadequate here and ringing people up, visiting them or short periods of secondment may be necessary to fill in the details. The transfer of research into practice also requires practitioners to have detailed knowledge about what actually happens in their own practice setting and what might be possible there (Chapter 8).

Research elsewhere is only the starting point of feasibility research in the local setting. As suggested in Chapter 5, action research can be an effective form of feasibility study: make a change and see what happens. But this is only so where there are minimal risks of harm arising from changing practice in such a speculative way. However, the term 'action research' is a slippery one. It is perhaps better to think of transferring research into practice as always involving an 'action research' *stage*. Just how much reading, planning, consulting and training comes before that should depend on how risky making the change is estimated to be.

One of the important local contextual factors identified in this chapter was resources. These are such an important matter in transferring research into practice that the next chapter is largely devoted to this topic and to questions of cost-effectiveness.

References

Anderson, D., Chenery, S. and Pease, K. (1995) *Biting Back: Tackling Repeat Burglary and Car Crime*, Crime Prevention and Detection Series, Paper 58, London, Home Office.

Bennett, T. (1991) 'The effectiveness of a police-initiated fear-reducing strategy', *British Journal of Criminology*, Vol. 31, pp. 1–14.

Berman, J. and Norton, N. (1985) 'Does professional training make a therapist more effective?', *Psychological Bulletin*, Vol. 98, pp. 401–7.

Bowling, A. (1997) *Research Methods in Health: Investigating Health and Health Services*, Buckingham, Open University Press.

Bucke, T. (1995) 'Policing and the public: findings from the 1994 British crime survey', *Research Findings*, No. 28, London, Home Office.

Buckley, R. and Caple, J. (1990) *The Theory and Practice of Training*, London, Kogan Page.

Brugha, T. and Glover, G. (1998) 'Process and health outcomes: need for clarity in systematic reviews of case management for severe mental disorders', *Health Trends*, Vol. 30, No. 3, pp. 76–79.

Burquest, R., Farrell, G. and Pease, K. (1992) 'Lessons from schools', *Policing*, Vol. 6, pp. 148–55.

Department of Health (1995) *Building Bridges: A Guide to Arrangements for Inter-Agency Working for the Care and Protection of Severely Mentally Ill People*, Wetherby, Department of Health.

Drury, W., Birchwood, M., Cochrane, R. and Macmillan, F. (1996a) 'Cognitive therapy and recovery for acute psychosis: a controlled trial. 1 Impact on psychotic symptoms', *British Journal of Psychiatry*, Vol. 169, No. 3, pp. 593–601.

Drury, W., Birchwood, M., Cochrane, R. and Macmillan, F. (1996b) 'Cognitive therapy and recovery for acute psychosis: a controlled trial. 2 Impact on recovery time', *British Journal of Psychiatry*, Vol. 169, No. 3, pp. 606–7.

Edgar, K. and O'Donnell, I. (1998) *Mandatory Drug Testing in Prisons: The Relationship between MDT and the Level and Nature of Drug Misuse*, Home Office Research Studies 189, London, Home Office.

Farrell, G. and Pease, K. (1993) *Once Bitten, Twice Bitten: Repeat Victimisation and Its Implications for Crime Prevention*, Crime Prevention Unit, Paper 46, London, Home Office.

Farrell, G., Phillips, C. and Pease, K. (1995) 'Taking like candy', *British Journal of Criminology*, Vol. 35, pp. 384–99.

Ford, R., Repper, J., Cooke, A., Norton, P., Beardsmoore, A. and Clark, C. (1993) *Implementing Case Management*, London, Research and Development for Psychiatry.

Forrester, D., Chatteron, M. and Pease, K. (1988) *The Kirkholt Burglary Prevention Project, Rochdale*, Crime Prevention Unit, Paper 13, London, Home Office.

Forrester, D., Frenz, S., O'Connell, M. and Pease, K. (1990) *The Kirkholt Burglary Prevention Project: Phase II*, London, Crime Prevention Unit, Paper 23, London, Home Office.

Gomm, R. (1996) *Co-ordinating Community Mental Health Care: The Care Programme Approach*, Milton Keynes, Social Services Inspectorate of the Department of Health/The Open University.

Hamblin, R. (1998) 'The wrong target', *Health Services Journal*, 2 April, pp. 28–31.

Howarth, I. (1989) 'Psychotherapy, who benefits?', *The Psychologist*, Vol. 2, No. 4, pp. 149–52.

Howe, D. (1987) *Introduction to Social Work Theory*, Aldershot, Wildwood House.

Howe, D. (1993) *On Being a Client: Understanding the Process of Counselling and Psychotherapy*, London, Sage.

Hunt, S. (1989) *Community Development and Health Promotion in a Deprived Area: Final Report*, Edinburgh, Research Unit in Health and Behavioural Change, University of Edinburgh.

Keep, J. (1998) 'Change management', in Bury, T. and Mead, J. (eds) *Evidence-based Healthcare: A Practical Guide for Therapists*, pp. 45–65, Oxford, Butterworth Heinemann.

Kemp, R., Hayward, G., Applethwaite, G., Everitt, B. and David, A. (1996) 'Compliance therapy in acute psychotic in-patients: a randomised control trial', *British Medical Journal*, Vol. 312, pp. 345–9.

Nutting, P. and Green, L. (1994) 'From research to practice: closing the loop in clinical policy development for primary care', in Dunn, E. V., Norton, P. G., Stewart, M., Tudiver, F. and Bass, M. J. (eds) *Disseminating Research/Changing Practice*, pp. 151–61, Thousand Oaks, Calif., Sage.

Pawson, R. and Tilley, N. (1997) *Realistic Evaluation*, London, Sage.

Sampson, A. and Phillips, C. (1992) *Multiple Victimisation: Racial Attacks on an East London Estate*, Crime Prevention Unit, Paper 36, London, Home Office.

Sapsford, R. and Abbott, P. (1992) *Research Methods of Nurses and the Caring Professions*, Buckingham, Open University Press.

Sechrest, L. (1994) 'Recipes for psychotherapy', *Journal of Consulting and Clinical Psychology*, Vol. 62, No. 5, pp. 952–4.

Sheldon, T., Guyatt, G. and Haines, A. (1998) 'When to act on evidence', *British Medical Journal*, Vol. 317, pp. 139–42.

Smith, M., Glass, G. and Miller, T. (1980) *The Benefits of Psychotherapy*, Baltimore, Johns Hopkins University Press.

Spinelli, E. (1994) *Demystifying Therapy*, London, Constable.

Stiles, W. (1994) 'Drugs, recipes, babies, bathwater and psychotherapy', *Journal of Consulting and Clinical Psychology*, Vol. 62, No. 5, pp. 955–9.

Tilley, N. (1993) 'Crime prevention and the Safer Cities story', *Howard Journal of Criminal Justice*, Vol. 32, pp. 40–57.

Tilley, N. (1996) 'Demonstration, exemplification, duplication and replication in evaluation research', *Evaluation*, Vol. 2, pp. 35–50.

Wright, L. (1999) 'Training needs analysis (TNA)', in Perkins, E., Simnett, I. and Wright, L. (eds) *Evidence-based Health Promotion*, pp. 91–98, Chichester, John Wiley and Sons.

Chapter 10
Should we afford it?

Roger Gomm

Introduction

When practitioners are thinking about applying research findings in practice they often have to address questions of cost. These are questions such as: 'What would it cost to do that?' or 'Would that cost be justifiable?' Costs might be monetary or in terms of client inconvenience, staff stress, and so on. They might be *opportunity costs*, which are the costs of not doing something desirable in order to do something else. Economic analyses attempt to answer questions about how much it costs to achieve something of value, or to avoid something undesirable (Jefferson *et al.*, 1996; Watson, 1997). Economic analysis is the topic of this chapter.

During the 1990s many health authorities established schemes to provide post-operative care in the patient's home rather than in hospital. A major motivation for these 'hospital at home' schemes was the assumption that they were more *cost-effective* than post-operative in-patient care. If so, this would mean that care of a quality equal to that provided for in-patients could be provided at home for a lower cost, or that care of a higher quality than in-patient care could be provided at home for the same cost. In this chapter, one such piece of research into the cost-effectiveness of a 'hospital at home' scheme is used as a case study.

This case study raises the issue of how much the preferences of patients are worth in terms of monetary costs to the NHS. For handling this kind of issue economists use the idea of *utility*. This is explained in Section 2 and illustrated by one of its most important applications in health care research: the Quality-adjusted Life Year or QALY. Earlier chapters drew attention to the problem of applying research findings about groups of people to decisions about individuals. *Decision analysis* is the economist's solution to this problem. This is explained in Section 3.

1　In-patient or hospital at home treatment?

The case study for this section is research done by Sasha Shepperd and several colleagues (Shepperd *et al.*, 1998a, b) comparing in-patient hospital care with hospital at home care (H-at-H). The latter means earlier discharge from hospital and the provision at home of services which would otherwise be provided in the hospital. These are services such as observation, administration of drugs, nursing care and rehabilitation. The study covered cases of hip replacement, knee replacement, hysterectomy, medical care for older people and chronic obstructive airways diseases. These cases are analysed separately since H-at-H might be cost-effective for some care groups and not for others.

According to a precise definition of terms, the researchers conducted a *cost-minimisation analysis* (Jefferson *et al.*, 1996, pp. 30–39). They compared two ways of achieving the same outcomes to find out which was cheapest. A *cost-effectiveness analysis* asks a slightly different question: 'Which of two ways of spending the same amount of money would produce the greatest benefit?' (Jefferson *et al.*, 1996, pp. 40–55). Although this is a different question, the kind of analysis used to produce the answer is essentially the same. Often the term 'cost-effectiveness' is used to refer to both analyses (Jefferson *et al.*, 1996, p. 52) and it will be used in the more inclusive way below. Whichever the question, both analyses have to start by comparing the effectiveness of different interventions, before considering issues of cost.

For this purpose, Shepperd *et al.* used a randomised controlled experimental design (see Chapter 3) with patients being allocated at random for in-patient or H-at-H treatment. Safety for discharge from hospital to H-at-H care and the suitability of home circumstances were threshold factors for inclusion in the trial, irrespective of to which arm of the trial people were allocated. Data were collected at the start, after one month and after three months (Shepperd *et al.*, 1998a).

The findings of the RCT were that:

> ... there are no major differences in patient assessed health outcomes between hospital at home and hospital care ... However, our results suggest that patients recovering from a knee replacement are not suitable for hospital at home care ... Although there were few differences in outcome, most patients preferred hospital at home care ... The preferences of carers were less strong than those of patients.
>
> (Shepperd *et al.*, 1998a, p. 1790)

This quotation concerns the effectiveness of treatments not their *cost-effectiveness*. Since, except for knee replacement patients, the two modes of treatment were more or less equally effective, the analysis then moves on to consider which could be provided at least cost:

> Many believe that hospital at home schemes will contain healthcare costs by reducing the demand for acute hospital beds. Our findings indicate that this is not the case. Instead, hospital at home care increased health service costs for some groups of patients, while for others there were no net differences in costs. ... The results of this trial suggest that simply shifting services from one location to another is unlikely to reduce health service costs.
>
> (Shepperd *et al.*, 1998b, p. 1795)

This second quotation claims that the expense of achieving similar outcomes was on average greater for H-at-H patients: that H-at-H was the less cost-effective option in terms of health service resource costs. But, putting those to one side, the H-at-H scheme seems to have been the most effective way of producing happy patients. There are issues here about how much extra the NHS should spend in order to produce patient satisfaction over and above, or irrespective of, the production of health gains measured more narrowly.

Outcome measurements

This is a cost-of-outcome study. Its findings depend on what outcomes were measured and how they were measured. There are three issues here for practitioners who read research:

1 Did the researchers use accurate and appropriate methods for measuring the outcomes they measured? Is the study believable in its own terms?

2 Were the outcomes they measured of the kind the reader would like to achieve in practice? Is the study relevant to the interests of the particular practitioner?

3 Does the study provide a clear indication for deciding between interventions?

Accurate and appropriate methods

The study used a wide variety of instruments to measure the health status of patients in terms of changes from base-line measurements, as appropriate to their main health problem. It used a carers' strain index to measure the burden on carers and a questionnaire to elicit preferred locations of care from carers and patients. The health measures included some that depended on the expert judgement of practitioners, but most measures asked patients to rate their own well-being, health, pain, competence in performing activities, and so on. There were no major discrepancies between self-assessments and assessments by practitioners.

Most of the instruments used had been validated for their validity and reliability (Jenkinson, 1994). Chapter 2 has an example of a questionnaire being subjected to this treatment (Cohen *et al.*, 1996) but not all such studies use well-validated instruments. Sometimes practitioner opinion is used as a basis for setting base-lines and measuring outcomes, without the aid of a standardised instrument. If different practitioners are involved as judges and decision-makers in the research, they may not make judgements in the same way as each other (Sackett *et al.*, 1991, pp. 35–39). Practitioner judgements do cause problems of interpretation in this study as regards judgements about when a patient should be discharged from H-at-H care. As discussed later in this section, different professional opinions about this have different cost implications.

Even well-validated instruments can produce misleading results in some circumstances. For example, many measurement scales show 'floor' and/or 'ceiling' effects (Wright, 1994, pp. 96–97). A scale measuring ambulatory function might do so only to the extent of giving the same score to all those who can walk. However, this may include some people who can just about walk and others who can run up stairs. The scale may score two treatments with similar outcomes. But the ceiling effect may hide the fact that one treatment has much better ambulatory outcomes than the other. Because they are designed to investigate illness and disability rather than health, all the major instruments for health and well-being self-assessment fail to discriminate between 'good' and 'excellent', and have a ceiling effect in this regard (Essink-Bot et al., 1997).

The research in question always entailed making comparisons between two groups (in-patient and H-at-H). But did each instrument measure the same attribute in both groups? For example, it is commonly observed that people move more confidently in their own homes than in strange environments. Do any differences between a hospital and an at-home population really show an ability to ambulate or, instead, confidence in ambulation? And would this matter? This issue does not seem to raise questions about the study by Shepperd et al. but it points towards some of the interpretive problems in reading this kind of research and applying it in practice.

The duration of a study will determine the outcomes that can be measured. The Shepperd study has a time frame of three months. If there were, say, a lower rate of readmission to hospital among the H-at-H patients after this, the conclusions about cost-effectiveness should be different from those published.

Are the outcome measurements relevant to the interests of other practitioners?

Someone reading the study by Shepperd et al. might be particularly interested in whether the in-patient or H-at-H experience enhanced the self-care skills of patients and carers and, if so, which did so most. They might be prepared to spend more on the option that was most successful in this respect. They would be operating with a different standard of effectiveness from the authors. This study would not give them the information they wanted, since the acquisition of self-care skills was not measured. Some areas of health and social care have great potential for different people to adopt different ideas of effectiveness, and hence to require different outcome measures. For example, in mental health, a study showing the cost-effectiveness of a drug in ameliorating schizophrenic symptoms (for example, Davies and Drummond, 1994) would not satisfy someone whose idea of effective mental health care was in terms of people learning to live with and to control their own symptoms with minimal medication and preferably no medication at all (Romme and Escher, 1993; Breggin, 1993).

Clear indications for decision making

A third important issue is about how to weight different outcomes, if one treatment rates better for one kind and the other for another kind of outcome. There might also be other relevant outcomes not measured by the study. The Shepperd study suggests that decision-makers will have to choose between two options, both more or less equivalent in producing health gains, but one being cheaper and less popular and one more popular and more expensive. At this point, cost-effectiveness/cost-minimisation analysis begins to drift into the area better dealt with by cost–utility analysis, which does have ways of dealing with such hybrid outcomes. This issue is picked up again in Section 2.

Measuring and assigning costs

The findings of many kinds of research are context-dependent (see Chapter 9, Figure 1). This is especially true of costs in economic research, since what it costs to achieve a particular outcome may be highly *sensitive* to local circumstances such as local wage rates, the seniority profile of an agency's staffing, the age and maintenance costs of buildings, split-site working and travelling distances. Any or all of the contextual factors identified in Chapter 9 may make what is cost-effective in one place less so, or more so, in another (Chapter 9, Tables 1 and 2). Also, factors like these can alter dramatically over short periods of time. For example, a cost-effective preference for a labour-intensive intervention, as opposed to a pharmaceutical one, can be quickly reversed if the patent on the drug of choice runs out and its price falls and/or if wages rise.

The results of economic analysis are also very sensitive to *how* costs are calculated. Table 1 (opposite) shows the costs for in-patient care compared with H-at-H for the hysterectomy patients only. The final row shows that the H-at-H scheme was more expensive by around £92 per patient. Since there were no significant differences in recovery between the two groups, this is the same as saying that in-patient recovery was the most cost-effective option. Note, however, that the only costs calculated here are health service costs.

The costing here is simply the average number of days of care (first four rows) each multiplied by the average cost per day of care, plus the average cost of GP services per patient. Thus for hospital care the average hospital cost per day was £111.88 (£647.77 divided by 5.79 days). The confidence intervals cited in the fourth column can be read as follows. A ratio of 1 would designate identical costs, so the ratio of 1.15 means that H-at-H is more expensive than in-patient care. A minus figure would have designated in-patient care as more expensive. The 95% confidence intervals (1.04 to 1.29) give a high degree of confidence that the difference is not just a matter of chance, since both limits are on the same side of 1.

Table 1   **Health service resources and costs consumed post-operatively for up to three months after hospital admission by patients allocated to hospital at home care or in-patient hospital care (patients recovering from hysterectomy)**

	*Hospital (123 patients)**	*Hospital at home (111 patients)†*	*Differences: H-at-H minus hospital (95% confidence intervals)*
Mean days in hospital care	5.79	4.34	–1.44 (–2.09 to –0.79)
Mean days in H-at-H care	–	3.11	–
Mean total days of care	5.79	7.45	1.66 (0.94 to 2.39)
Median (interquartile range) days of readmission‡	0.00	0 .00	P = 0.21 (Mann–Whitney U test)
Mean hospital costs including readmission‡	£647.77	£487.43	Ratio of geometric mean 0.76 (0.67 to 0.87) P<0.01
Mean H-at-H costs	–	£250.18	–
Mean (inter-quartile range) GP costs: home and surgery visits	£30.98 (15.49–61.96)	£30.98 (15.49–61.96)	P = 0.70 (Mann–Whitney U test)
Mean total health service costs	£679.39	£771.78	Ratio of geometric mean 1.15 (1.04 to 1.29) P<0.01

* No data available for one patient.
† No data available for three patients.
‡ There were no readmissions to hospital for hysterectomy patients.

(Source: based on Shepperd *et al.*, 1998b, p. 1793)

Some insight into the costing can be gained from the following quotation, which refers to costing H-at-H:

> The costs of nurses, physiotherapists, and occupational therapists were based on the amount of time spent with patients, and included a cost for non-contact time. The following non-staff costs were included: central administration, travel, training, telephones and pagers, equipment, and office space. Medical supplies and equipment costs were depreciated over a 10 year period with a discount rate of 6%. These costs were apportioned on an equal basis to each patient receiving hospital at home care, assuming costs were payable in advance at the start of the year.

> Administration and travel costs were apportioned according to the volume of patients. The cost of prescribed drugs was obtained from the hospital's pharmacy department.
>
> (Shepperd *et al.*, 1998b, p. 1792)

Different ways of calculating costs in cost-effectiveness analyses can result in different figures, and sometimes different conclusions. Unlike financial accountancy in general, there are no standard conventions for accountancy in cost-effectiveness studies (Jefferson *et al.*, 1996). Two things to look for are:

- transparency – whether the authors explain how costs were calculated
- even-handedness – since comparisons are being made, were the costs for one mode of intervention calculated in the same way as for the other?

Here, for example, if the hospital costs had included a consideration for the capital depreciation of the hospital buildings, while the GP costs included no consideration for the capital depreciation of their surgeries, this would spuriously depress the cost of the H-at-H scheme for groups visited frequently by the GP, such as the obstructed airways patients cared for by H-at-H. In fact, in this study something like the reverse happened. Since GPs were paid extra for visiting patients in this demonstration project, this increased the cost of H-at-H compared with the costs that would have accrued had they been accommodated within normal GP practice budgets. Interventions involving different mixes of services from different agencies often give rise to problems of costing, since hospitals, general practices, social services departments, and so on all keep their accounts and do their costings in different ways.

Sometimes a short cut is taken. The actual number of days or episodes of care may be counted but then they are costed from nationally or regionally averaged data. The Policy Studies Research Unit at the University of Kent, for example, regularly publishes indicative costings for primary care and social services (for example, Netten and Dennet, 1996). Averaged health services costs are available for each nation of the UK through regional offices of the NHS. When this short cut is taken, the results must be read with an 'if' in front: *if* the costs were indeed as for the standardised costs *then* ... (Whynes and Walker, 1995). However, this does not matter much for the person thinking of using a published cost-effectiveness analysis to inform a local decision elsewhere. Here the important cost data are the local ones, not those in the research study, and the real local ones, not indicative ones produced from averaging costs across different institutions and departments.

The job of calculating the costs is done better by an accountant or a finance officer than by most health and social care practitioners; further sources of advice are Yates (1996), Smith and Wright (1994), Netten and Beecham (1993) and Clark and Lapsley (1996).

What costs are counted in the research is an important matter. They may include costs that are not relevant to making a local decision elsewhere, and they may exclude costs that are relevant. For example, a scheme that looks highly cost-effective in the research may not be so somewhere else if implementing it means purchasing new buildings or refurbishing old ones. These will be real costs against the scheme.

Whose costs is also an important question. In the study by Shepperd *et al.*, financial costs to carers were calculated. They were greater for the H-at-H scheme but negligible when averaged over all clients. This was because there was little in the way of loss of earnings, most carers being retired. Non-financial costs were also calculated, using a stress measurement scale for carers, and showed little difference between the two schemes.

The cost-for-whom question comes up in another guise. Shepperd *et al.* do not cost for home care services provided by social services. Many cost-effectiveness studies are institutionally bounded like this. An agency can increase its own cost-effectiveness by cost shunting: making sure that another agency picks up the tab or cares for the most expensive clients. In this case, however, it is a good guess that adding in costs to social services would have made H-at-H look even less cost-effective.

The *when* of costs can also be important. For example, at one time minor tranquillizers looked cost-effective but their addictive qualities made them very costly in the long run (Gabe, 1996). The practice of discounting in economic analyses (see the quotation above) recognises that money spent now might have generated an income later and resources consumed may have to be replaced at higher prices (Sheldon, 1992).

What works for whom?

In the study by Shepperd *et al.* clients were randomly allocated to in-patient or H-at-H care. It is fairly certain that the higher cost of H-at-H was not due to the sicker patients being allocated to H-at-H. This also means that the results of this study tell of the relative cost-effectiveness of the two treatments *when clients are allocated to them at random.*

But the question practitioners want answered is different. It is: 'Would it be most cost-effective to have a hospital at home scheme just for those most suitable for that?' and there is the ancillary question: 'Could we, in practice, successfully allocate the clients to the scheme most appropriate for them?'

At least some of the additional costs of H-at-H seem to arise from allocating to it patients who developed complications and would have been better, and more cheaply, dealt with had they been in-patients. Knee-replacement patients, for example, showed high average H-at-H costs because they were so frequently readmitted to hospital because their replacement broke down. Shepperd *et al.* conclude that this shows H-at-H is not cost-effective for knee-replacement patients in general. But H-at-H

might be cost-effective for just those knee-replacement patients least likely
to suffer from breakdown. An intervention which shows poor *average*
outcomes may none the less be the best treatment, and the most cost-
effective one, for a minority. If that minority can be identified then it may
be possible to increase overall cost-effectiveness by providing this option
for them alone: by *targeting* treatment. Thus, if it could be predicted in
advance who would be high-cost H-at-H patients, they could be allocated
to in-patient treatment, and the cost-effectiveness of H-at-H would
improve.

Reliability of practitioner judgements

To accept the findings of the Shepperd study fully, it has to be assumed that,
wherever they received their care, both patient groups were served by
equally effective staff, who made judgements in the same way as each other.
The researchers themselves raise an issue here. Depending on the client
group, H-at-H patients were on average receiving between one-and-a-half
and nine more days of treatment than the in-patients. Was the additional
cost of H-at-H due to staff spending more time with these patients than was
necessary to produce the same outcomes as for the in-patient group? The
possibility is accommodated for in one of the several sensitivity analyses
done by the researchers.

Sensitivity analysis

Economic analysts are well aware that their findings relate to just a
particular state of affairs at a particular time. Therefore, they often do
sensitivity analyses. These are 'What if?' calculations: for example, 'What
if nurses' salaries rose relative to other costs?'; 'How high would nurses'
salaries have to rise for the option using most nurse time to cease to be the
more cost-effective?'

Given their concern that H-at-H staff might be spending longer than
necessary with their patients, Shepperd *et al.* did the sensitivity analysis in
Table 2 (opposite).

This analysis *does not* show that H-at-H would be more cost-effective if
less time was spent with H-at-H patients. It *does* show that it would be
more cost-effective *if* less time were spent *and if* the same outcomes were
achieved as in the trial. The study was not designed to investigate the
effect of varying the time spent with patients, so this sensitivity analysis
raises an issue without resolving it. This is not always so with sensitivity
analyses. In studies of the cost-effectiveness of pharmaceuticals, for
example, once the relative effectiveness of two drugs has been established
through an RCT, ready-reckoners can be drawn up showing the threshold

Table 2   **Sensitivity analysis of relative costs of in-patient care and hospital at home care with varying average length of hospital at home treatment (hysterectomy patients only)**

Varying assumption	Cost per case of H-at-H above or below cost of in-patient care
Average time as actually recorded	+£92.40 (H-at-H is more expensive than in-patient care)
Estimate if H-at-H was on average one day shorter than the time actually recorded	–£21.75 (H-at-H would be cheaper than in-patient care)
Estimate if H-at-H was on average two days shorter than the time actually recorded	–£80.48 (H-at-H would be much cheaper than in-patient care)

(Source: based on Shepperd *et al.*, 1998b, p. 1794)

prices at which it would be more *cost*-effective to prescribe one drug rather than another (for example, Duggan *et al.*, 1998; Delaney and Hobbs, 1998).

The trial involved paying GPs extra for their involvement in the study. Shepperd *et al.* also did a sensitivity analysis varying the cost of GP services. Cost-effectiveness for the hysterectomy patients was *not* sensitive to GP costs, since the H-at-H patients were visited no more often than the in-patients post-discharge (see Table 1). Changing the costs of GP care would affect in-patients and H-at-H patients equally. But the H-at-H obstructed airways patients were visited much more often by GPs than their in-patient counterparts. If, instead of being paid extra, GPs had to accommodate these costs within their ordinary practice budget, the H-at-H costs for obstructed airways patients would fall more than the costs for the in-patients.

But this, in turn, raises other cost questions for an agency wanting to implement its own H-at-H scheme: 'Who would bear the costs of GPs spending more time with more H-at-H patients?'; 'Is there money to pay GPs for taking on work which would otherwise be done by hospital doctors, or would the costs appear as GP time lost by other patients or by GP over-work?'; and 'Would the GPs be willing to participate?' This is one of those 'institutional structure' questions raised in Chapter 9.

Feasibility and commitment

The community nursing staff for H-at-H patients were special appointees, probably pleased to be involved in an interesting research project. They may have spent more time with the patients as a result (Sapsford and Abbott, 1992, p. 105). This may have pushed up the cost of H-at-H. But making a rule to limit the numbers of days of care given at home could not be done without undermining the clinical freedom of community nurses and GPs. Steve Illiffe, commenting on this study, suggests that characteristics of the institutional structure might also be at play:

> Were hospital at home teams having difficulty discharging patients, perhaps with perverse incentives to hold on to them during periods of underutilisation? Or is discharge from inpatient care sometimes premature, so that recipients of hospital at home services get longer, but more appropriate, care?
>
> (Illiffe, 1998, p. 1761)

Even if assessment techniques were available to avoid allocating inappropriate patients to H-at-H, or there were protocols determining when people should be discharged, would practitioners use them? And what about patient choice? In practice, it is actually very difficult to compel practitioners to make decisions on a cost-effective basis, even assuming that there is evidence available to tell them what is the most cost-effective decision to make in each instance.

National and local decision making and cost-effectiveness analysis

The Shepperd study is one of several economic analyses of hospital at home schemes conducted after a large number of schemes had been set up. Some of these analyses show H-at-H schemes to be the more cost-effective (Knowelden *et al.*, 1991; O'Cathain, 1994; Coast *et al.*, 1998); some (Hensher *et al.*, 1996), as Shepperd *et al.*, the less cost-effective. But these are different schemes, with different clients, in areas with different cost structures and using different costing methodologies and somewhat different outcome measures. It would be dangerous, therefore, to take any one of them as the basis for making national policy (Illiffe, 1997, 1998). Because cost-effectiveness is so sensitive to local circumstances, local circumstances should determine local policy, and the important economic analysis is a local one.

This does not mean that such studies have no wider interest. A study such as that by Shepperd *et al.* provides a model which can be tweaked to fit local circumstances elsewhere and into which local costings can be substituted for the ones used by the researchers. What is transferable from such research is not so much the findings as the methodology.

2　Cost–utility studies

In the study by Shepperd *et al.* the production of patient satisfaction ran in the direction opposite to the cost-effective production of health gains whether measured objectively or subjectively. If there is not much difference between two treatments in terms of health gains, perhaps patient preferences should be allowed to decide the issue. Since this would result in a more costly service, this consideration raises the question of how to put a value on giving patients what they would find most satisfactory.

For economists, *utility* is a measure of satisfaction (Torrance, 1986). Thus a *cost–utility* study calculates the cost of producing a unit of satisfaction. For the H-at-H scheme, how much would it cost to give each patient the care location of their choice?

Utilities are always someone's utilities. Different decision-makers may make different choices. These choices will depend on the institutional structure within which they make decisions. For example, Shepperd *et al.* analyse the H-at-H scheme in terms of costs to the NHS in a way that is abstracted from the realities of NHS budgetary decision making. Within the NHS different costs fall on different budgets. The study was done at a time of GP fund-holder purchasing. Then an important issue would have been the question of how much extra GPs would be willing to pay NHS trusts in order to give their patients the option of H-at-H. This is rather different from giving GPs sweeteners to participate in the study. By the time the study by Shepperd *et al.* was published, the institutional structure for decision making had changed with the advent of Primary Care Groups (Primary Care Co-ops and Primary Care Trusts in Scotland).

Quality-adjusted Life Years

Quality-adjusted Life Years (QALYs) are the most important example of utility measures used for research and decision making in health care (Bowling, 1991, 1997), although they would not be very useful for making decisions about a hospital at home scheme.

QALYs bring into the same scheme of measurement the 'hard' indicator of life expectancy and the more qualitative, or 'soft', notion of quality of life (QOL). The QALY measurement was introduced as a remedy for the crude practice of judging medical interventions just in terms of the (easily measurable) number of additional years of life they achieved, without taking account of the fact that such extra years might be of very variable quality. Too enthusiastic a pursuit of survival rates would lead to large numbers of people being maintained on life-support machines, or alive but severely disabled by heroic medical intervention.

Figure 1 (overleaf) shows one component of the ED-5DQ questionnaire developed Europe-wide for surveying the self-rated health of populations. It is sometimes used to provide an outcome measure in RCTs. Other experimental research and similar scales were used in the H-at-H study. The same device is also used as a basis for assigning values to different states of health, relative either to death or to 'perfect health', thus serving as utilities in cost–utility analysis (EuroQol Group, 1990; Kind *et al.*, 1998; Watson, 1997, pp. 138–41).

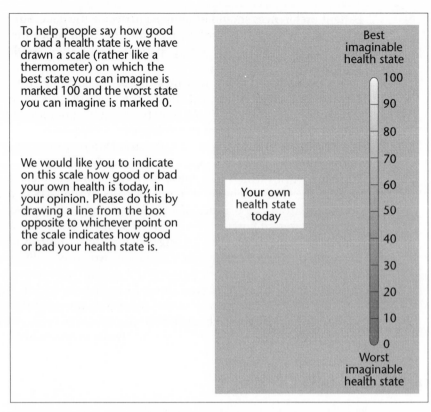

To help people say how good or bad a health state is, we have drawn a scale (rather like a thermometer) on which the best state you can imagine is marked 100 and the worst state you can imagine is marked 0.

We would like you to indicate on this scale how good or bad your own health is today, in your opinion. Please do this by drawing a line from the box opposite to whichever point on the scale indicates how good or bad your health state is.

Best imaginable health state

100
90
80
70
60
50
40
30
20
10
0

Your own health state today

Worst imaginable health state

Figure 1   **Quality of life (QOL) measurement instrument taken from a EuroQol questionnaire** (Source: Kind *et al.*, 1998, p. 740)

There are at least five different ways of calculating QALYs, which give rather different results (Richardson, 1992, pp. 40–41; Torrance, 1986), and many QALY-like alternatives (Bowling, 1991). As a starting-point they all involve eliciting from people their preference for living in a disabled or an uncomfortable state rather than death. This yields a utility (satisfaction measure) in the form of a quality of life measurement or QOL. Then cost–utility studies can be used to determine the costs of improving quality of life as measured in this way. The simplest device for eliciting QOLs is the so-called 'straight line method'. Someone is presented with a line, running from 1 through 0, where 1 is a state of perfect health and absence of disability and 0 is death (see Figure 1). Some people will regard death as the worst possible state of health. Others will regard being kept on a life-support machine as worse than death. Alternatively, or as well, people can be asked how much less than perfect health they would regard, for example, blindness: perhaps scoring that at 0.75 if they thought blindness was one-quarter short of perfect health. The result of this kind of scoring is QOL scores such as those in Table 3, which are group averages in this case.

Table 3 **QOL scores for various states of health and disability: average scores elicited from various samples of people**

Health state	Utility value* (QOLs)
Healthy (reference state)	1.00
Life with menopausal symptoms	0.99
Mild angina	0.90
Kidney transplant (rated by transplant patients)	0.84
Moderate angina	0.70
Hospital dialysis (rated by dialysis patients)	0.57
Hospital dialysis (rated by general public)	0.56
Severe angina	0.50
Anxious/depressed and lonely much of the time	0.45
Being blind, deaf or dumb	0.39
Needing mechanical aids to walk and learning disabled	0.31
Dead (reference state)	0.00
Quadraplegic, blind and depressed	Less than 0.00
Unconscious	Less than 0.00

*May also be expressed as percentages (1.00 = 100%)

(Source: based on Torrance, 1987, cited in Richardson, 1992, p. 25)

These are QOLs and not yet QALYs but they are a basis for calculating them. QALYs draw in addition on the survival curves expressing the life expectancy of people of different ages with different medical conditions, with or without treatments of particular kinds. Then the following kind of calculation is done.

Suppose, for example, that a particular patient group has a condition QOL-rated at 0.85 and they have an average life expectancy of 15 years. An operation is available that will improve their rating from 0.85 to 0.97 *and* increase average life expectancy to 17 years.

Without operation	*With operation*
15 years more life	17 years more life
@ 0.85	@ 0.97
= 12.75 QALYs	= 16.49 QALYs

A subtraction shows that, on average, each operation generates an extra 3.74 QALYs.

Now suppose that this operation costs £2000 per patient on average, net of savings in care costs consequent on improving the patient's condition and/or of increased costs consequent on them living longer. A question that can now be asked is whether there is an alternative way of spending £2000 per head on this patient group which will achieve more than 3.74 QALYs each; or, alternatively, whether there is a way of achieving 3.74 QALYs per head at less than £2000 per head. Unless there is some very good reason for deciding otherwise, the preferred treatment is the one that produces most extra QALYs per unit of cost. This is the most cost-effective treatment in QALY terms.

QALY calculations are often used in making resource allocation decisions where different options for expenditure differ markedly in cost and/or life expectancies and/or life quality. With the establishment in 1999 of the National Institute for Clinical Excellence (NICE) in England, Wales and Northern Ireland and its Scottish equivalent, QALYs are likely to feature even more prominently in future. The function of these bodies is to produce national guidelines on cost-effective practice.

All resource allocation decisions in public services are controversial (New and Le Grand, 1996). One of the advantages of using QALYs in making health care rationing decisions is that the way they are calculated can be made completely transparent, so that decisions can be queried and critiqued more easily than decisions based on whim, political compromise or historical inertia (Watson, 1997). Of course, the results of QALY calculations depend on whose QOL ratings are entered into the equation. As might be guessed, the rating of 'being blind, deaf or dumb' (Table 3) at 39% 'perfect health' was not derived from the opinions of blind, deaf or dumb people. But whichever decisions are made, and however they are made, they are based on someone's values (Harris, 1987). Using QALYs forces this out into the open because it is necessary to specify whether the QOL ratings came from patients, representative samples of the public or practitioners.

3   Chances, choices and expected utilities

QALYs and similar utilities can also be used to make decisions about individual patients, where the patient's *own* quality of life ratings are used to calculate the best value option. Chance then becomes an important factor, as follows.

The average life expectancy of a large group of people with other known characteristics can be calculated with great precision but this cannot be done for any one of them in particular. Thus, while a group might have an average life expectancy of four years after an operation, it may not be known which individuals among them will live longer or less than this

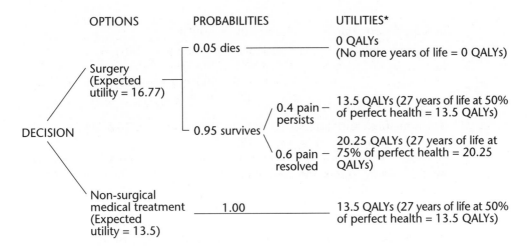

OPTIONS   PROBABILITIES   UTILITIES*

0.05 dies — 0 QALYs
(No more years of life = 0 QALYs)

Surgery
(Expected
utility = 16.77)

0.4 pain persists — 13.5 QALYs (27 years of life at 50% of perfect health = 13.5 QALYs)

DECISION

0.95 survives

0.6 pain resolved — 20.25 QALYs (27 years of life at 75% of perfect health = 20.25 QALYs)

Non-surgical
medical treatment   1.00 — 13.5 QALYs (27 years of life at 50% of perfect health = 13.5 QALYs)
(Expected
utility = 13.5)

* The doctor estimates that, operative risk apart, this patient can expect to live for 27 years. Using a straight-line method the patient may have rated death at zero, life with pancreatitis but without pain at 75% (0.75) of perfect health, and life with pancreatitis and pain at 50% (0.5)

Figure 2 **A decision tree for calculating the expected length of quality-adjusted life for two treatments for chronic pancreatitis** (Source: based on Bursztajn et al., 1990, p. 219)

(Gould, 1998). Also, not only is post-treatment life expectancy unpredictable, so too is post-treatment (and post-non-treatment) quality of life.

Decision analysis extends economic analysis to take account of chance, including cost–utility analyses using QALYs (Dowie, 1996; Lilford et al., 1998). Figure 2 shows the kind of decision tree that features in this kind of analysis.

In this example, costs to the health service are not considered. The costs and benefits considered are those impacting on the patient. The patient's own ratings of health were used to produce the quality of life component (the QOLs) of the QALY scores – perhaps using the 'straight line method' described in Section 2, together with expert estimations of life expectancy for someone of the patient's age and medical condition, with or without the operation. The decision is whether to have a surgical operation or to continue with non-medical treatment. This is not a straightforward decision since surgery entails a 5% risk of death – shown as a probability of 0.05 on the decision tree. Moreover, even if the patient survives the operation, there is only a 60% (0.6) chance that the pain will be relieved. The patient may end up after the operation with the same life expectancy and the same dismal quality of life as before. The probability figures will be derived from research findings tweaked by the clinician to fit the particular circumstances of this patient.

The calculations necessary to identify the best value choice are simple. They go as follows.

For surgery [first branch]   (Probability × utility) +

[second branch]   Probability ((Probability × utility) +
                                  (Probability × utility))

$$= (0.05 \times 0) + (0.99((0.4 \times 13.5) + (0.6 \times 20.25)))$$
$$= 0 + (0.99(5.4 + 12.15))$$
$$= 17.37$$

For non-surgical treatment there is a 100% chance of 13.5 QALYs, so the calculation is simply $1 \times 13.5 = 13.5$.

These two figures (17.37 and 13.5) are called *expected utilities*. The highest figure offers the best chance of achieving the most desirable outcome. In this case the surgical operation is the best bet. Because the decision has to be made under conditions of uncertainty, gambling is unavoidable. The patient may opt for surgery and die from the operation, but the chances of a successful outcome instead, and the strength of the patient's preference for a pain-free life, seem high enough to justify taking this risk compared with the alternative of non-surgical treatment.

Increasingly, this kind of calculation is being built into computer software designed as 'decision aids' for clinicians who have to help patients make an informed choice about their own treatment. These are usually in a ready-reckoner form showing what decision should be made according to the preferences (utilities) expressed by the patient on the one hand and the risks (probabilities) for this particular patient on the other (Bursztajn *et al.*, 1990; Dowie, 1996).

Decision analysis is not confined to life-and-death matters nor to utilities expressed as QALYs. Indeed, its most common application is in business risk assessment. Wherever making a decision entails uncertainties – which is true of most decisions – decision analysis can be used to identify the 'best bet' option.

Conclusion

Practices and forms of organisations are never just cost-effective or cost-ineffective. Any set of practices is amenable to a wide range of judgements according to what costs are taken into consideration, what benefits are counted against the costs, on whom costs fall and to whom benefits accrue; and according to who does the valuation and who says what counts as 'effective'. There are no right answers in economic analysis but its procedures make the standards and the process of judgement explicit.

The findings of economic analyses are often highly sensitive to local contextual factors determining costs, whether these are expressed in money terms or in terms of staff stress or client dissatisfaction; and to local factors determining outcomes, for example staff expertise, or the peculiarities of an agency's client mix. Under some circumstances the findings of an economic analysis will be robust and widely generalisable. This will be where the costs and the benefits are uniform, or can be made uniform across different agencies and localities, and the intervention is a simple one and not sensitive to differences in practitioner expertise. Economic analyses of immunisation programmes and some health-screening programmes come close to this (Stewart-Brown, 1997). Even here the findings are vulnerable to cost changes over time, and to therapeutic developments that replace yesterday's best value practice with today's.

Most practices in health and social care are much more context-dependent than immunisation or screening programmes. Thus published economic analyses can rarely be taken to apply directly to anywhere other than the locale in which they were done, at the time they were done. None the less, they are useful for practitioners working somewhere else because they provide a model for a local economic analysis, substituting local costs and local preferences for those in the research study. Even if a practitioner's local version may be a somewhat ramshackle and speculative affair, the costings are almost bound to be more accurate for the local situation than research in a situation elsewhere.

Cost-minimisation and cost-effectiveness analyses (narrowly defined) do not necessarily exclude qualitative matters such as the clients' preferences or their own feelings of well-being. Indeed, most of the outcome measures in the RCT done by Shepperd *et al.* were self-assessments by clients. But it is much easier to accommodate client preferences in cost–utility analyses. Adding decision analysis can put the clients in the driving seat by helping them to clarify what choices are available to them, how much they want one outcome more than another and what risks are associated with particular choices. In bringing research evidence (the probabilities) together with client preferences (the utilities), decision analysis allows for research evidence to be applied at the level of the individual client.

References

Bowling, A. (1991) *Measuring Health: A Review of Quality of Life Measures*, Buckingham, Open University Press.

Bowling, A. (1997) *Research Methods in Health: Investigating Health and Health Services*, Buckingham, Open University Press.

Breggin, P. (1993) *Toxic Psychiatry: Drugs and Electroconvulsive Therapy – The Truth and Better Alternatives*, London, Fontana.

Bursztajn, H., Feinbloom, R., Hamm, R. and Brodsky, A. (1990) *Medical Choices, Medical Chances: How Patients, Families and Physicians Can Cope with Uncertainty*, London, Routledge.

Clark, C. and Lapsley, I. (eds) (1996) *Planning and Costing Community Care*, London, Jessica Kingsley Publishers.

Coast, J., Richards, S., Peters, T., Gunnell, D., Darlow, A.-M. and Poundsford, J. (1998) 'Hospital at home or acute hospital care? A cost minimisation analysis', *British Medical Journal*, Vol. 316, pp. 1802–6.

Cohen, G., Forbes, J. and Garraway, M. (1996) 'Can different patient satisfaction survey methods yield consistent results? Comparison of three surveys', *British Medical Journal*, Vol. 313, pp. 841–44.

Davies, L. and Drummond, M. (1994) 'Economics and schizophrenia: the real cost', *British Journal of Psychiatry*, Vol. 165 (Supplement 25), pp. 18–21.

Delaney, B. and Hobbs, F. (1998) 'Commentary: *Helicobacter pylori* eradication in primary care', *British Medical Journal*, Vol. 316, p. 1654.

Dowie, J. (1996) 'The research-practice gap and the role of decision analysis in closing it', *Health Care Analysis*, Vol. 4, pp. 5–18.

Duggan, A., Tolley, K., Hawkey, C. and Logan, R. (1998) 'Varying efficacy of *Helicobacter pylori* eradication regimes: cost effectiveness study using a decision analysis model', *British Medical Journal*, Vol. 316, pp. 1648–54.

Essink-Bot, M.-L., Krabbe, P., Bonsel, G. and Aaronson, N. (1997) 'An empirical comparison of four generic health status measures', *Medical Care*, Vol. 35, No. 5, pp. 522–37.

EuroQol Group (1990) 'EuroQol – a new facility for the measurement of health-related quality of life', *Health Policy*, Vol. 16, pp. 199–208.

Gabe, J. (1996) 'The history of tranquilliser use', in Heller, T., Reynolds, J., Gomm, R., Muston, R. and Pattison, S. (eds) *Mental Health Matters: A Reader*, pp. 186–95, Basingstoke, Macmillan.

Gould, S. J. (1998) 'The median isn't the message', in Greenhalgh, T. and Hurwitz, B. (eds) *Narrative Based Medicine: Dialogue and Discourse in Clinical Practice*, pp. 29–33, London, BMJ Books.

Harris, J. (1987) 'QALYfying the value of life', *Journal of Medical Ethics*, Vol. 13, pp. 117–23.

Hensher, M., Fulop, N., Hood, S. and Ujah, S. (1996) 'Does hospital at home make economic sense? Early discharge versus standard care for orthopaedic patients', *Journal of the Royal Society of Medicine*, Vol. 89, pp. 548–51.

Illiffe, S. (1997) 'Hospital at home: buyer beware!', *Journal of the Royal Society of Medicine*, Vol. 90, pp. 181–2.

Illiffe, S. (1998) 'Hospital at home: from red to amber?', *British Medical Journal*, Vol. 316, p. 1761.

Jefferson, T., Demichelli, V. and Mugford, M. (1996) *Elementary Economic Evaluation in Health Care*, London, BMJ Publishing Group.

Jenkinson, C. (ed.) (1994) *Measuring Health and Medical Outcomes*, London, UCL Press.

Kind, P., Dolan, P., Gudex, C. and Williams, A. (1998) 'Variations in population health status: results from a United Kingdom national questionnaire survey', *British Medical Journal*, Vol. 316, pp. 736–41.

Knowelden, J., Westlake, L., Wright, K. and Clarke, S. (1991) 'Peterborough Hospital at Home: an evaluation', *Journal of Public Health Medicine*, Vol. 13, pp. 182–8.

Lilford, R., Pauker, S., Braunholtz, D. and Chard, J. (1998) 'Decision analysis and the implementation of research findings', *British Medical Journal*, Vol. 317, pp. 405–9.

Netten, A. and Beecham, J. (eds) (1993) *Costing Community Care: Theory and Practice*, Aldershot, Ashgate.

Netten, A. and Dennet, J. (1996) *Unit Costs of Community Care 1996*, Canterbury, Personal Social Services Research Unit, University of Kent.

New, B. and Le Grand, J. (1996) *Rationing in the NHS: Principles and Pragmatism*, London, King's Fund.

O'Cathain, A. (1994) 'Evaluation of a hospital at home scheme for the early discharge of patients with fractured neck of femur', *Journal of Public Health Medicine*, Vol. 16, pp. 205–10.

Richardson, J. (1992) 'Cost–utility analyses in health care: present status and future issues', in Daly, J., McDonald, I. and Willis, E. (eds) *Researching Health Care: Designs, Dilemmas, Disciplines*, pp. 21–44, London, Routledge.

Romme, M. and Escher, S. (1993) *Accepting Voices*, London, Mind.

Sackett, D., Haynes, R., Guyatt, G. and Tugwell, P. (1991) *Clinical Epidemiology – A Basic Science for Clinical Medicine*, London, Little, Brown and Co.

Sapsford, R. and Abbott, P. (1992) *Research Methods for Nurses and the Caring Professions*, Buckingham, Open University Press.

Sheldon, T. (1992) 'Discounting in health care decision-making: time for a change?', *Journal of Public Health Medicine*, Vol. 14, pp. 250–56.

Shepperd, S., Harwood, D., Jenkinson, C., Gray, A., Vessey, M. and Morgan, P. (1998a) 'Randomised controlled trial comparing hospital at home care with inpatient hospital care. I: three month follow up of health outcomes', *British Medical Journal*, Vol. 316, pp. 1786–91.

Shepperd, S., Harwood, D., Gray, A., Vessey, M. and Morgan, P. (1998b) 'Randomised controlled trial comparing hospital at home care with inpatient hospital care. II: cost minimisation analysis', *British Medical Journal*, Vol. 316, pp. 1791–96.

Smith, K. and Wright, K. (1994) 'Informal care and economic appraisal: a discussion of possible methodological approaches', *Health Economics*, Vol. 3, pp. 137–48.

Stewart-Brown, S. (1997) 'Evaluating screening programmes: theory and practice', in Jenkinson, C. (ed.) *Assessment and Evaluation of Health and Medical Care: A Methods Text*, pp. 151–70, Buckingham, Open University Press.

Torrance, G. (1986) 'Measurement of health state utilities for economic appraisal: a review', *Journal of Health Economics*, Vol. 5, pp. 1–30.

Torrance, G. (1987) 'Utility approach to measuring health-related quality of life', *Journal of Chronic Diseases*, Vol. 40, No. 6, pp. 593–600.

Watson, K. (1997) 'Economic evaluation of health care', in Jenkinson, C. (ed.) *Assessment and Evaluation of Health and Medical Care: A Methods Text*, pp. 129–50, Buckingham, Open University Press.

Whynes, D. and Walker, A. (1995) 'On approximations in treatment costing', *Health Economics*, Vol. 4, pp. 31–39.

Wright, L. (1994) 'The long and the short of it: the development of the SF-36 General Health Survey', in Jenkinson, C. (ed.) *Assessment and Evaluation of Health and Medical Care: A Methods Text*, pp. 89–105, Buckingham, Open University Press.

Yates, B. (1996) *Analyzing Costs, Procedures, Processes and Outcomes in Human Services*, London, Sage.

Chapter 11
Evidence for planning services

Roger Gomm

Introduction

Many planning decisions have to be made several years in advance because they involve capital investments or organisational changes or because there is a bidding procedure where bids take a long time to prepare and process. To design services appropriately, it is necessary to use evidence that is available now in order to make predictions about some future state of affairs. The kinds of evidence considered in this chapter include demographic evidence, epidemiological evidence, evidence drawn from services as they are operating now, evidence from research elsewhere and evidence from local surveys and consultation events.

1   A Single Regeneration Budget bid as an example

This chapter features a Regeneration Partnership preparing a bid under the terms of the Single Regeneration Budget (SRB) scheme. The details are fictional but based on the author's experience of three real SRB bids. SRB is an example of 'challenge' funding awarded through a competitive bidding process. City Challenge, Safer Cities funding, Health Action Zones, Education Action Zones, Drug Action Challenge funding and Early Years Partnership funding are similar examples.

This example has five features that are even more general.

1 *A short lead time*. Being able to work from a good pre-existing database puts a bidding partnership at an advantage.

2 *Collaborative bidding*. Bidders here were a partnership including: local government (two tiers, and in the roles of housing, education, social services, probation, police, planning and environmental health authorities); health (health authority and NHS trust); the police; local industry and commerce; the Training Enterprise Council; the chamber of local employers; and voluntary sector agencies.

3 *A requirement for public and service-user consultation*. For most schemes, central government specifies consultation in particular with minority ethnic groups and other 'hard-to-reach' sections of the population, such as disaffected young people. For schemes delivering a service, consultation with actual or potential service-users is usually required.

4 *A requirement for the plans to be co-ordinated with other local polices and strategies.* Here this included a housing investment programme (HIP), the local Children Plan, a Community Care Plan under Section 42 of the National Health Service and Community Care Act 1990, Health Improvement Programmes (HImPs), Drug Action planning under the Tackling Drugs Together strategies, and other local policies.

5 *Matched funding.* For every pound awarded by central government, local agencies have to guarantee expenditure of their own. What percentage depends on the scheme concerned. Such schemes have to be carefully costed (see Chapter 10).

The SRB case also illustrates the importance of evidence about 'deprivation' in determining funding by central government.

In brief, putting together an SRB bid meant the following.

- Identifying an area of the town as 'deprived' and giving evidence of its deprivation.
- Through multi-agency collaboration, thinking up good ideas for ameliorating its deprivation.
- Consulting with the publics of the identified area about their concerns and preferences.
- Whittling down the ideas to just those that were affordable; those for which evidence could be produced of their likely effectiveness; and those for which evidence could be produced of local demand.
- Planning to implement these ideas in conjunction with other relevant local plans, which meant getting the objectives and the finance for the SRB bid written into, for example, the Housing Investment Plan and the Community Care Plan.
- Costing the plans, and giving undertakings that local agencies would match the funding provided by central government.
- Providing evidence that the bid had been produced through a collaborative and consultative process.
- Establishing performance targets and monitoring systems.

There were at least 10 collaborative meetings involving 156 people from 17 different agencies, many small groups in between, and four episodes of public consultation. There were another four consultation events involving minority ethnic groups, two special events for young people, and a house-to-house survey. The real cost of preparing the bid was around £65,000. The bid failed. However, the partnership was successful in a later round of bidding, with a somewhat different plan. Much of what featured in the original plan was put into operation in other ways with other monies. Two years later almost the same partnership – although with a different name – engaged on a bigger collaborative activity in drawing up the local crime and disorder audit and strategy as required by the Crime and Disorder Act 1998. Much of the groundwork for this had already been accomplished in terms of evidence collection and in brokering collaborative relationships between agencies. The original bid failed but the planning did not.

2   Demographics, deprivation and epidemiology

Demographic evidence

All service planning has to begin with evidence about the kinds of people who live in the planning area: their age, gender, ethnic group, socio-economic status; how many of each, and so on. Many of the demographic data used for local planning either derive directly from the 10-year national censuses or are updates of census data (Dale and Marsh, 1993) (see Box 1).

Box 1: Decennial census data relevant to local health and social care planning

- Numbers of people by age, sex, ethnicity, country of birth, marital status, type of employment, educational level, house tenure, housing quality, overcrowding, household composition, car ownership, journey to work, limiting and long-standing illness.

- Available for small areas (Enumeration Districts and electoral wards), for local government areas, and for health authority/board districts, areas and regions (in Northern Ireland for Health and Social Services Board areas), regionally and nationally. There are separate censuses for England and Wales, Scotland and Northern Ireland.

- There are also mid-decade 10% sample censuses. These do not collect information about everyone but they do provide information about population trends to correct the broader features of the local demographic picture.

Despite the problem of dating, census data are still usually the best basis for building a model of the local population that will represent the up-to-date situation. 'Building a model' means mainly making some guesstimates and tweaking the census data to update them in the light of whatever other evidence is available (Field and MacGregor, 1987).

Other routinely collected information can be used to make estimates of change locally. These include, for example, data deriving from the registration of births and deaths, on school rolls, and on welfare benefits and data kept by housing authorities (Unwin *et al.*, 1997). The annual exercise of registering electors provides some (albeit incomplete) information about the numbers and genders of adults. Some local authorities use the same mailing (which they must do by law) as an opportunity to do a mini-census of their own.

All District, Borough, Shire and Unitary authorities and all health authorities/boards (in Northern Ireland, Health and Social Services Boards) have some kind of statistical service which maintains an up-to-date demographic model for their area. For the SRB bid the authority had to make population projections for five years hence on the basis of census data that were five years out of date.

Both the County Council and the District Authority had their own demographic model for the town as a whole and its population of around 80,000. But the SRB bid was for a cluster of adjoining wards in the town: a population of around 12,000. The larger the population unit, the less accurate the figures need to be for planning. In an area the size of Belfast, an extra 200 five-year-olds spread across the city is neither here nor there in planning terms. But if they all unexpectedly arrived in one ward of the city that would be a different matter. Four reasons make it difficult to give accurate estimates for small areas, unless they are so small that it is feasible and affordable to collect the information directly.

1   Except in rare circumstances, the 10-year census is the only occasion when detailed information is collected from every household. Between censuses the smaller the area, the more out of date the statistics.

2   Much routinely recorded information – births, deaths, unemployment rates, crime rates, and often information about the use of services – cannot be linked to a small area without needing a special exercise, and it is given for a whole town and/or the health authority district or area. Data about the patients of a GP practice, or about a secondary school, or about the clients of a Community Drug and Alcohol Team, do not necessarily refer to coterminus areas. With the advent of postcodes and computerised record keeping this is becoming less of a problem, since client postcodes can be linked to the census areas (Noble and Smith, 1994).

3   After the birth rate, geographical mobility is the most difficult factor to estimate (Field and MacGregor, 1987). Much is short-range – to another 'small area' within the same town. Individual wards may increase or decrease dramatically in population, change their age structures radically, become deprived or gentrified, or change their ethnic mix, while the size, age, socio-economic and ethnic profiles of the larger population remain the same or change in a different way.

4   Most *ad hoc* social survey work is based on drawing samples from an area much bigger than a ward. A sample which is representative for a town will not necessarily provide sound evidence for making decisions about any of its smaller divisions.

The authorities involved in the SRB bid could give an accurate picture of the demographics of the town as a whole but there was less certainty about the age, gender and ethnic structure of the wards featured in the bid. As the lead authority was a housing authority, it could fill in the picture from its knowledge of its own council-house tenants and its nominees for housing-association property. Together these made up 45% of households.

Deprivation formulae

Central government financing for local spending is adjusted according to the socio-economic circumstances of an area, because poorer populations have more of the kinds of problems with which health and social care services deal. Deprivation is usually defined by *deprivation indices* (sometimes called under-privileged area or UPA scores). The score on such an index was crucially important in the SRB bid. The more deprived an area was, the more likely the bid was to be successful.

Deprivation *indicators* are both easily measured and associated with deprivation or affluence. Deprivation *indices* are single scores derived from combining several indicators. The index score locates an area on a scale from 'extremely deprived' to 'extremely affluent'. Areas can then be ranked in 'league tables' of deprivation.

In allocating health service monies, the first deprivation indicator used in this way (from 1976) was simply the standard(ised) mortality ratio (SMR), which is a measure of how far the death rate of an area departs from the national death rate, after discounting for the differences in age structures between areas (Unwin *et al.*, 1997, pp. 28–35). Before this, health service money was distributed largely on a historic basis. Since there had always been more health service provision in the more affluent (and healthier) south-east of England, this area got a disproportionate share of the funds. Using the SMR as a deprivation, or need, indicator redistributed resources to poorer areas with their higher death rates, although in the face of enormous opposition from those areas, which saw their incomes growing more slowly than in the areas of greater gain. The Conservative government of 1993 wanted to match NHS expenditure to deprivation much more closely and used a deprivation formula devised at the University of York (Judge and Mays, 1994). In 1999, modifications of this were still the basis on which central government health funding was adjusted to take account of deprivation.

The Standard Spending Assessment for England, and similar formulae for other parts of the UK, determines central government funds for local authority expenditure. Again deprivation indicators are involved. This applies also to the social services expenditures of the Northern Ireland Health and Social Services Boards, and the education expenditures of the Northern Ireland Education Board. Numbers of young people are also an important component of the calculation here, for obvious reasons. Box 2 shows the English Department of the Environment, Transport and the Regions' *Index of Local Deprivation* for 1998 – a slightly different version from the *1991 Index of Local Conditions* (Department of the Environment, 1994) which applied to the SRB bid.

The Department of the Environment in England, and the equivalent departments of the Scottish, Welsh and Northern Ireland Offices, also maintain deprivation league tables of local authority areas based on such deprivation indicators. A high score on all or most indicators puts an area somewhere towards the top of the deprivation league table.

The deprivation indices noted above are used as administrative devices. For research purposes it is more usual to use either the Jarman-10 or the Jarman-8 Index (Jarman, 1983) or the Townsend Index (Townsend *et al.*, 1985, 1988). Different indices are appropriate for different purposes. For example, the Jarman Index is used to weight payments to GP practices

---

Box 2: Index of Local Deprivation 1998 – the 12 indicators*

1 *Unemployment rate* (1997 Office of National Statistics)

2 *Housing lacking amenities* (1991 census)

3 *Overcrowded housing* (1991 census)

4 *Dependent children of income support recipients* (1996 DSS data)

5 Non income support recipients in receipt of Council Tax Benefit (1996 DSS data)

6 Low educational participation aged 17 (1991 census)

7 Low educational attainment (percentage of 15-year-olds gaining GCSE passes at grades D–G only, plus those not gaining any GCSE passes) (1996 DfEE)

8 Standard mortality ratios for under-75s (1996 Office of National Statistics) – double weighted

9 Home insurance weightings (1996) (insurance companies – proxy for extent of crime victimisation) – double weighted

10 Derelict land (1993 DoE)

11 Male long-term unemployment (1997 Office of National Statistics)

12 Number of beneficiaries on income support (DSS 1996)

*The indicators in italics are available at ward/enumeration district level and local authority district level; the others at LA district level only.

(Source: adapted from DETR, 1998, pp. 11–12)

---

because it includes proportions of children under five, pensioners living alone, and recent immigrants, which add to the workload of a GP practice, although not necessarily to an area's deprivation (Porteous, 1996, p. 33).

Sometimes people regard this kind of measurement with great suspicion. But if they were pressed to be precise about what they meant by saying that one area was more 'deprived' than another, the only satisfactory answer they could give would look rather like an exercise in selecting deprivation indicators and scoring areas in these terms.

Indicators and indexes are 'objective': not necessarily true but at least transparent. If someone disagrees with an index figure, at least they know what it is they are disagreeing with. Because they are transparent in this way, deprivation indicators allow for different areas to be compared on a common standard. Some kind of redistributive equity can be achieved by directing more resources to areas with higher index figures or, in the case of SRB bids, by prioritising bids from areas with the highest deprivation scores. Different ways of calculating such indexes have benefits for some areas and disadvantages for others, often measurable in tens of millions of pounds. They are often queried by authorities who believe that a different way of calculating deprivation would be 'fairer'. A particularly common complaint from rural areas is that *at local authority level* these indices are blind to rural poverty, which is often hidden in small pockets in otherwise affluent areas (Abbott *et al.*, 1993).

As Box 2 shows, only a few deprivation indicators relevant to the SRB bid are available at the level of small areas. Three of them are based on very out-of-date information. In making their bid, the SRB Partnership could also point to some indicators of deprivation that are not used in government formulae. These included crime victimisation maps from the police, and the Citizen's Advice Bureau's estimate of the number of people from the identified area seeking help with debt. As the lead agency was the authority administering housing and council tax benefits, it could provide up-to-date data on these for the wards in question.

Epidemiological research

The justification for using deprivation indices depends on how far a measure of deprivation can be used to predict the extent of illness or social problems. Put another way, deprivation indicators are *validated* by seeing how well the index predicts what is known about illness and social problems in areas where the extent of illness and social problems is known. If the index survives this test, it can be used with some confidence to estimate the extent of illness or social problems in areas where these are *unknown* (for example, Jarman *et al.*, 1992). A good index *discriminates* between areas so that the higher the deprivation score, the higher the burden of illness or social problems, step by step along the scale.

Validating a deprivation index relies on epidemiological research. Medical epidemiology is a large field of research, but its major preoccupation is with detecting the patterns taken by diseases, asking who is most likely to get what disease and under what circumstances (Unwin *et al.*, 1997; McConway, 1994). Although the term 'epidemiology' may not be used, people who study social problems are often engaged in the same kind of enterprise. There is an epidemiology of crime (Anderson *et al.*, 1995), racial harassment (Sampson and Phillips, 1992), child abuse, and any field where 'risk factors' are identified.

The two major objectives of epidemiological research are, first, to discover what causes what, and hence how it can be prevented or treated. So, for example, what really does cause new strain CJD? Second, and more modestly, it aims to discover what is regularly associated with what, as a step towards working out the cause, but also as a way of predicting which kinds of people are most at risk, say, of contracting HIV or of being a victim of burglary, or which areas are most likely to have the highest rates of child accidents or high rates of mental illness, or which occupational groups show high risks of testicular cancer.

It is better to know *how* a problem is caused. However, simply being able to predict *who* is most likely to suffer from it is useful in making decisions about deploying resources or targeting health education.

Epidemiology was introduced with a prior discussion of deprivation indices because most illnesses, most forms of disability and most social problems show a close relationship with deprivation (Benzeval *et al.*, 1995).

One of the starkest ways of demonstrating this is by mapping. The maps in Figure 1 (overleaf) show the ranking of wards in Sheffield according to a deprivation index. The eight most deprived wards include the seven with the highest death rates and the five with the highest rates of admission to mental hospital. There would also have been a close correlation between the ranking for deprivation and ranking in terms of the percentages of babies born with low birth weights.

While many conditions particularly afflict older people or minority ethnic groups or women or men, the poorer they are, the more they are at risk. For example, sickle-cell anaemia is largely restricted to people with African ancestry, and thalassaemia to people with a Mediterranean ancestry, but the prognosis depends to some extent on the past and current deprivation of the person carrying the gene concerned (Smaje, 1995). For most kinds of illness, however, socio-economic status rather than ethnicity seems to be a more important factor (Nazroo, 1997a, pp. 107–9; 1997b).

Deprivation indicators are useful general-purpose tools for predicting levels of physical and mental health or levels of community stress *in general*. They are far less useful for predicting the incidence of any *particular* disease or social problem in an area. Medical epidemiology produces estimates of the prevalence and incidence of most major diseases (Unwin *et al.*, 1997). It would be prohibitively expensive for each health authority to conduct firsthand research into the extent and distribution of all the diseases in its own area. Hence, local health service planning has to rely to a considerable extent on extrapolating from studies done somewhere else from the local circumstances.

Since 1991 the NHS Management Executive (1991) has commissioned many Health Care Needs Assessment Reviews. These collate what is known about the geographical and social distribution of particular medical conditions to produce models of the prevalence of the condition that might be expected in a notional health district of around a quarter or half a million people (Stevens and Raftery, 1994, 1997). Prevalence is how many people in a given population will be suffering from the condition at a particular time. These models have to be adjusted according to the characteristics of real-life areas. For example, if the disease is age-related, such as Alzheimer's disease, then the model will have to be adjusted in the light of the local age profile (Meltzer, 1992). If, as is usually the case, the disease shows a pattern related to deprivation, estimates for the local area will need to be adjusted accordingly. Data from the census and particularly from the General Household Survey provide the basis for estimating the

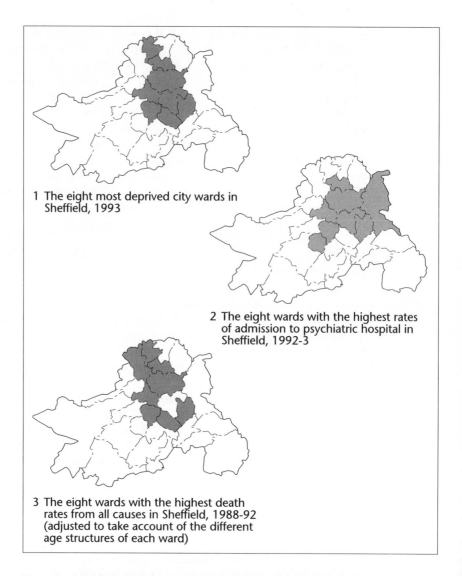

1 The eight most deprived city wards in Sheffield, 1993

2 The eight wards with the highest rates of admission to psychiatric hospital in Sheffield, 1992-3

3 The eight wards with the highest death rates from all causes in Sheffield, 1988-92 (adjusted to take account of the different age structures of each ward)

Figure 1   **Social deprivation, mortality and psychiatric admissions in Sheffield** (Source: Sheffield Health, 1994, unpublished)

extent of 'limiting and long-term' illness in local areas (Kind *et al.*, 1998), while the British Crime Survey provides data that are useful for building local models of crime victimisation and drug abuse (for example, Mirrlees-Black, 1998; Mirrlees-Black and Byron, 1998). As with demographic models, it is easier to produce accurate models for larger rather than smaller populations (Williams and Wright, 1998, p. 1381).

Local predictions like these will become increasingly important with the further development of primary care group, health 'co-op' or primary care trust commissioning. Currently, the performance indicators for primary care handed down from central government (NHS Executive, 1998) take little account of the socio-economic circumstances of different areas (McColl *et al.*, 1998). It would be more sensible to judge performance in primary care in terms of success in reducing disease *below* the figure predicted by the local demographic and socio-economic situation. The same would be true for performance indicators for Community Safety Partnerships and Drug Action Teams, since crime, accidents, drug addiction, alcoholism, child abuse and domestic violence all show a close association with social deprivation and population age profiles.

For the SRB bid, the prevalence of particular illnesses turned out not to be an important issue. Early attempts to produce an epidemiological profile of the SRB wards with local data from GP and health-visiting records proved fruitless. The population was registered with a large number of practices and the practice actually in the area had many patients drawn from other areas. The information technology in use did not allow for automated analysis (see Chapter 8). This reflects the current state of agency record-keeping. But, increasingly, agencies are acquiring electronic recording systems with a GIS capacity (Local Government Management Board, 1994; Noble and Smith, 1994). Geographical information systems can map cases to postcodes, allowing:

- an agency to investigate the geographical pattern of its own cases and services (see Box 3 overleaf)
- an agency to map its current cases against deprivation maps provided by the Office of National Statistics (in terms of the deprivation indicators referred to earlier)
- cases from many agencies to be displayed on a common map.

The maps of crime victimisation featured in the SRB bid were produced with the police GIS. These showed the wards concerned as 'hot spots' for burglary, street robberies, disturbances and domestic assaults.

However, GISs are only as good as the local data entered into them.

3   Service data and research on effectiveness

Service data

Health, housing, social care and criminal justice agencies generate huge quantities of data: about the characteristics of their clients, about interventions made and their outcomes. Such data enter into epidemiological research and into making planning decisions (Brown, 1996; Foreman, 1996; Percy-Smith, 1996).

Box 3: Geographical information about demand for child care in Oldham

To produce the map in Figure 2 the GIS mapped the residence of all children under four living in families dependent on benefit *and* all available child-care places, play-groups, nurseries and registered child-minders. It then calculated the number of child-care places within a 'pram-push' of each child's home: up to 1000 metres, or up to a major barrier such as a busy road. The two kinds of data were then mapped on to each other to produce the map in Figure 2, showing those areas with shortages of 20 full-time equivalent places or more.

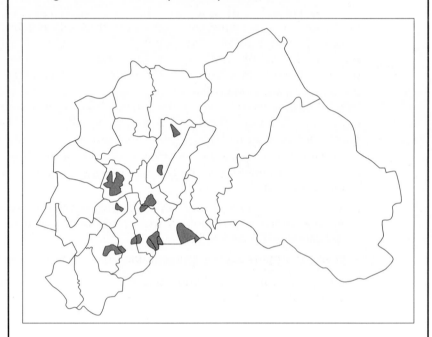

Figure 2   **Areas with excess demand over supply of child care places** (Source: Noble and Smith, 1994, p. 373)

This can be very important evidence but there is one particular problem with it. The evidence generated in the course of delivering a service is primarily evidence about how service organisations work. In Chapter 7 there is an example of how data on the number of dilatation and curettage operations in Buckinghamshire reflected idiosyncratic decision making within and between NHS trusts, rather than the pattern of conditions remediable through D&Cs (Holton and Needham, 1995). If the interest is epidemiological, there is a grave danger that service data will tell not about the epidemiology of an illness but about the epidemiology of seeking treatment and being processed through a health care system (White *et al.*, 1961). Service data will only tell about the people the service is actually dealing with, and not about those to whom it is inaccessible.

Correcting service data is often difficult. If services on the ground could not find 'missing' potential service-users, how can researchers do so? One possibility is to use social survey techniques to get an estimate of under- or overuse of services by particular groups of people. In epidemiology, the term 'community survey' implies using survey research to find cases of illness *irrespective* of whether they are known to treatment agencies (for example, Nazroo, 1997a and b). Box 4 gives an example of an epidemiological health needs assessment, which used a community survey to check whether services were being targeted at those who needed them most.

Box 4: Example of an epidemiological health needs assessment

Objective: To assess whether the use of health services by people with coronary heart disease reflected need.

Setting: Sheffield health authority with a population of 530,000.

Methods: The prevalence of angina was determined by a validated postal questionnaire. Routine health data were collected on standardised mortality ratios; admission rates for coronary heart disease; and operation rates for angiography, angioplasty, and coronary heart disease. Census data were used to calculate Townsend scores to describe deprivation for electoral wards. Prevalence of angina and use of services were then compared with deprivation scores for each ward.

Results: Angina and mortality from heart disease [were] more common in wards with high deprivation scores. Treatment by revascularisation procedures was more common in more affluent wards.

Conclusion: The use of revascularisation services was not commensurate with need. Steps should be taken to ensure that health care is targeted at those who most need it.

(Source: Williams and Wright, 1998, p. 1382, citing Payne and Saul, 1997)

Community surveys are extremely expensive and they are rarely mounted solely to inform practice in just one local area. Rather, community surveys are used to provide information to estimate how much the service data from a local area are likely to be under-recording the prevalence of some condition in many areas. A clear example of this is the use of the British Crime Survey to provide estimates of the extent to which crime in a local area underestimates the true level of crime (Bottomley and Pease, 1986).

For some purposes a simple check can be made of the demographic characteristics of the people using a service as against a demographic model of the catchment area (Blackman, 1995). If there are no epidemiological reasons to explain things otherwise, mismatches probably indicate groups that find it difficult to access services. This has been a common strategy for studying service use by members of minority ethnic groups (Smaje, 1995). Another approach is to observe the way in which services are accessed and how practitioners make decisions. If these processes are understood, some judgements can be made about the accuracy of the data they generate (Gephart, 1988).

Another kind of service data that was important for the SRB bid was information about costs, which is discussed throughout Chapter 10.

Evidence from effectiveness research

The SRB bidders had to propose ideas that looked as if they would have the desired effects. For this they needed to consult and cite research studies on the effectiveness of intervention programmes. Chapters 9 and 10 discuss the possibilities and problems of basing action in one area on research done elsewhere. The SRB bid developed a strong law-and-order slant. In their bidding the partnership cited the research evidence on the effectiveness of closed-circuit television surveillance, environmental modification to reduce crime, property marking and 'target hardening'. Some of these are considered in Chapter 9. The bidders would have been wise to cross-map this research evidence against local conditions, as that chapter suggests. In fact, they merely assumed that if something worked somewhere else, it would work in their area. Indeed, they assumed it would produce results cost-effectively too, which is usually a rather cavalier assumption (see Chapter 10).

4   Asking people questions

The SRB bid involved four kinds of asking:

- asking practitioners, service managers and members of organised service-user and community groups – mainly by involving them in the bidding process
- asking 'the public' by holding public consultation events
- asking 'the public' through a sample survey
- asking young people through a survey designed and conducted by a group of young people resident in the area.

Public consultations

Unless they relate to a 'hot' political issue, hardly anyone will go to public consultation events. There is a widespread reluctance to participate in public affairs in general (Cooper *et al.*, 1995). There is also a problem in that people do not necessarily see themselves as part of 'the public' at which a public consultation event is aimed. The turn-out is better at consultation events aimed specifically at groups people do think they belong to: for example, as parents of children at the local school, or as members of the local Urdu-speaking community. Thus the best way of going through the motions of public consultation by having open meetings is also the best way of making sure that consultation is with very unrepresentative sections of the public: with the movers and shakers, the already organised and the more articulate people. The public consultation meetings associated with the SRB bid were poorly and almost exclusively attended by members of the two small local residents' associations, who were also the core of Neighbourhood Watch, by representatives from church congregations (who worshipped but did not live in the area) and by members of the town's Ethnic Minorities Forum, who also had four consultation meetings just to themselves. This was despite a flyer being delivered to every household in the area, a double-page spread in the local free newspaper, the events being featured on local radio, all known organisations being written to and asked to announce the events and publish them in their newsletters, and pamphlets and posters being displayed in community centres, newsagents, surgeries, pubs, betting shops and rent offices.

By contrast, the consultation meetings arranged specifically for members of minority ethnic groups were well attended – over-attended in fact, since many who came did not live in the SRB areas. The special meetings arranged for young people traded on the near-captive audience of the local youth club. From this a smaller group of young people did their own, rather haphazard survey of young people's opinions.

Citizen juries and focus groups

Two techniques the SRB partnership *did not* set out to use were *focus groups* and *citizen juries*. These both involve convening groups of people. With a citizen jury the group is presented with expert evidence. As with a trial jury, the members are asked to make a decision but here, perhaps, about which services a health authority should commission. A consensus view is expected to emerge. Citizen juries are quite commonly used as an adjunct of health and social care planning (McIver, 1998). But, unlike in Oregon in the USA, in the Netherlands and in parts of Germany, the jury never actually makes the final decision in the UK. Here it is probably appropriate to regard citizen juries as an extension of the 'lay-member' principle so widely used in decision-making bodies in health and social care.

Focus groups, by contrast, are recorded group discussions, without any decision making, and no consensus view is expected (Krueger, 1994; Barbour and Kitzinger, 1999). The attendance at the public consultation events was so low that they actually turned out rather like focus groups, with their attendant disadvantage of not being representative of a wider population. The latter criticism is also often levelled at citizen juries (McIver, 1998, p. 76). Data collected in group situations also have the disadvantage of being influenced by whoever are the higher status or the more assertive participants (Conning *et al.*, 1997; Green and Hart, 1999). For example, in SRB consultations with minority ethnic groups, the Bangladeshi participants usually looked to their imam for a lead. However, focus groups have also been said to provide a supportive environment in which people will feel more comfortable than in one-to-one interviews and, hence, more likely to say what they really think (Chiu and Knight, 1999). Using 'naturally occurring' groups as if they were focus groups is a common way of reaching otherwise hard-to-reach people, and has often been used as a community work approach to judging their opinions (Jowell *et al.*, 1990).

Focus groups are also commended for the richness of the data they generate (Krueger, 1994), by contrast with the data collected from questionnaires. However, for the purposes of the SRB bid, the partnership did not want rich, meaningful data showing the complexity of local opinion and subtle differences of viewpoint. It is difficult to see what they could have done with such data had they obtained them. What they wanted was a simple picture of what most concerned the majority of people living in the designated wards, and of the kinds of projects they would find most acceptable.

Surveys and representativeness

Public consultation events, focus groups and citizen juries are rarely representative of the wider public but properly designed sample surveys can be (see Chapter 2).

The SRB survey used a systematic sample with streets of the relevant areas as the 'sampling frame' or starting point. Thus every tenth house was selected. The units of sampling were residences, not people. Anyone aged 18 or over who answered the door and/or agreed to participate was selected. Resources allowed for one call back, at a different time of day from the first try in order to minimise non-response, and for a call back with an interpreter if necessary. The non-response was only 18%, which is good for house-to-house surveys.

Allowing anyone at an address to respond to a questionnaire is a departure from best practice in sampling because people who answer the door at a particular time of day will not be a representative sample of the population. There are techniques for randomly selecting household members without prior knowledge of household composition (Kish, 1965) but the survey team did not use them. Without prior knowledge of the ethnic composition of the area, they did not stratify by ethnicity (see Chapter 2, Section 1).

All surveys need to ask some questions to allow for the estimation of the representativeness of the respondents. So this survey included a question each on age, gender and ethnicity and a question on whether the property was council, housing association or privately owned. The survey team did not know for sure what the age, sex and ethnic composition of the area *as a whole* was but it did have accurate data on these characteristics for the adult population of public sector housing. Thus it was able to compare the questionnaire returns from public sector housing for age, sex and ethnicity with similar data from the housing records. In so far as there were discrepancies, these provided a direct estimate of the unrepresentativeness for public sector tenants, and an indirect and more speculative estimate for the owner–occupiers. On this basis they concluded that the survey was representative as regards the public/private distinction, that it over-represented older people (they were the ones who were usually at home) and, hence, under-represented minority ethnic people (who were younger on average). But among minority ethnic people the sample over-represented younger people – probably because they were the English-speakers called to deal with a stranger at the door. Also, because of the small numbers, the sample was not representative of the range of age groups *within particular* minority ethnic groups.

So, the SRB survey sample was not entirely representative but then few are. However, the majority responses in the survey were so clear that this really did not matter. The function of the survey was not to produce a fine-grained picture of diversity but to serve as a plebiscite: a way of testing majority opinion in the community about priorities. In exercises such as this, minority opinions, while interesting, are not the important issue. The survey first asked people to rank what they saw as the problems of the area from a given list. Overwhelmingly, people placed crime and vandalism as either the worst or the second worst problem: 72% of respondents gave these ranks. This preference held across ages, genders and ethnicities. Limited employment prospects was the nearest competitor. Then respondents were asked to complete the sentence 'What this area needs most is ...'. The responses here were what might have been predicted from the first part of the survey. But this did generate some ideas about interventions that might be welcomed locally: for example, 'more police on the beat', 'more powers for the police to deal with hooligans', 'community workshops', 'job creation', 'better street lighting'.

In these respects the survey gave the same results as the consultations with the general public. The consultation events with minority ethnic people had a rather different flavour. Law and order was still at the top of their agenda but more was said about racially motivated crime and about racist graffiti rather than graffiti in general. What no one had predicted was the concern with domestic violence in minority ethnic households. Even though this showed up on the crime victimisation maps produced by the police, it was not on the questionnaire, so there was no way of knowing whether this was also an important concern of the majority population, or among members of minority ethnic groups not participating in the consultations. Focus groups, and similar consultation formats, often throw up issues that are missed by questionnaire research and pose a puzzle about whether these are issues of importance just to the people in the focus group or more generally. The capacity of focus groups to generate issues (rather than answers) is one of the reasons why they are sometimes used as a preliminary to questionnaire research. The former helps to design the questions; the latter serves as a defence against letting the unrepresentative opinions of a small group of people determine decisions that will affect many others (Conning *et al.*, 1997).

Consultation with young people revolved around the youth club and involved a detached youth worker working with young people on the street. A group of four or five young people designed their own questionnaire, administered it according to methods that are not entirely clear, and gave a verbal report on the result to a group of councillors. They reported on the need for better youth facilities, and on grievances about being picked on by the police, scapegoating, and so on. In terms of research methodology, their research left almost everything to be desired. But, as often happens in participatory research of this kind, the prime purpose was not to produce accurate and representative statistical data but to give those involved a sense of having a stake in the exercise, to offer them opportunities to develop and exercise skills, and so on.

Constructing the need for services

The survey results were the reason why the SRB bid took such a strong law-and-order line. The plan that emerged featured proactive policing, a shop-front advice agency with drug advice and victim support, and a minority ethnic advocacy worker and detached youth workers to deal with the most troublesome young people. There was to be some environmental engineering to improve community safety, a project to help parents deal with 'out-of-control' children and a localised 'welfare-to-work' service. If the survey had turned out differently, the bid might have featured improved health services, or improved housing stock, a women's resource centre, a neighbourhood social work office, a credit union, or something different. All these were early ideas floated by agencies collaborating in the planning process.

At first sight the bid looks like a straightforward conversion of local demand into a plan for a local package of services. But what could be demanded was already shaped. The survey limited expressions of concern to those on a given list. The whole exercise was limited to considering services that could be provided at small area level. The respondent who suggested what the area most needed was for the UK to leave the European Community misunderstood the nature of the exercise. Similarly, the aggregation of demand always depends on the constituencies involved. Had the survey been directed only at single parent families, for example, a different set of second-order priorities would probably have emerged. Or people living in smaller areas within the small areas might have ranked preferences differently from each other. A wide and diverse constituency tends to overwhelm the demands of minority groups within it.

Asking people to put their demands in priority order and then calculating majorities is essentially a voting procedure. Votes go to majorities. If the survey had not asked respondents to put their preferences in rank order but merely to express their concerns, someone would have had to impose a priority order for the purpose of making a decision about which to respond to. If that privileged a minority it would be regarded as undemocratic. If it privileged a majority it would be critiqued as failing to respond to the needs of minorities. Survey or no survey, planners are often in a no-win situation.

There is also a problem with developing services as a rapid response to public demand. Planning here was for two years hence. Two years later much the same set of partner agencies did a community safety audit as required by the Crime and Disorder Act 1998. Only crime and community safety issues were relevant. Among these an issue appeared at the top of the public priorities that was not mentioned by anyone in the SRB surveys and consultations. This was the issue of 'dangerous paedophiles' and a demand for local measures to protect children from them.

Conclusion

Local firsthand research is extremely expensive. This chapter drew attention to the importance for local purposes of making use of whatever data are collected nationally or from elsewhere. Demographic and epidemiological models derived from this can then be adjusted in the light of local evidence. Much of the local evidence will come from service data. The limitations of such data have been noted. But, as suggested throughout Chapter 8, service data will always be the most important source of locally collected evidence.

This chapter was about evidence for making decisions that would affect large numbers of people. It would be grossly inequitable to base such decisions on the views of unrepresentative minorities and here a sample survey was the most appropriate method for gathering information about local views. Inevitably, sample surveys collect rather superficial data. In gathering evidence for making decisions affecting only a few people, in-depth interviews, a focus group or participant observation research might have been feasible and appropriate (see Chapter 4). It is important to distinguish between using research to gather evidence and using research as a means of community or personal development (Chapter 5). For the latter purpose, the level of involvement achieved is as important as the quality of the evidence produced. Research with a high level of participation almost inevitably involves only a few people.

'The public' or 'service-users' are not necessarily the best judges of what is feasible, or of what would be effective interventions. As Ann Bowling (1993) points out, the kinds of health services that would arise if they exactly met the majority priorities of the public would be very different from the kinds that research evidence suggests would generate the greatest health gains. Whatever the field of health and social care, evidence of public demand has to be tempered with evidence about what are effective (Chapter 3) and cost-effective (Chapter 10) provisions, and with the knowledge that public opinion can often be fickle.

References

Abbott, P., Bernie, J., Payne, G. and Sapsford, R. (1993) 'Health and material deprivation in Plymouth', in Abbott, P. and Sapsford, R. (eds) *Research into Practice: A Reader for Nurses and the Caring Professions*, pp. 129–55, Buckingham, Open University Press.

Anderson, D., Chenery, S. and Pease, K. (1995) *Biting Back: Repeat Burglary and Car Crime*, Crime Prevention and Detection Series, Paper 58, London, Home Office.

Barbour, R. and Kitzinger, J. (eds) (1999) *Developing Focus Group Research: Politics, Theory and Practice*, London, Sage.

Benzeval, M., Judge, K. and Whitehead, M. (1995) *Tackling Inequalities in Health: An Agenda for Action*, London, King's Fund.

Blackman, T. (1995) *Urban Policy in Practice*, London, Routledge.

Bottomley, K. and Pease, K. (1986) *Crime and Punishment: Interpreting the Data*, Milton Keynes, Open University Press.

Bowling, A. (1993) *What People Say About Prioritising Health Services*, London, King's Fund Centre.

Brown, M. (1996) 'Needs assessment and community care', in Percy-Smith, J. (ed.) *Needs Assessment in Public Policy*, pp. 49–65, Buckingham, Open University Press.

Chiu, L.-F. and Knight, D. (1999) 'How useful are focus groups for obtaining the views of minority groups?', in Barbour, R. and Kitzinger, J. (eds) *Developing Focus Group Research: Politics, Theory and Practice*, pp. 99–112, London, Sage.

Conning, S., Fellowes, D. and Sheldon, H. (1997) 'Users' views in theory and practice', *Journal of Clinical Effectiveness*, Vol. 2, No. 2, pp. 31–34.

Cooper, L., Coote, A., Davies, A. and Jackson, C. (1995) *Voices Off: Tackling the Democratic Deficit in Health*, London, Institute for Public Policy Research.

Dale, A. and Marsh, C. (eds) (1993) *The 1991 Census User's Guide*, London, HMSO.

Department of the Environment (1994) *The 1991 Index of Local Conditions*, London, HMSO.

Department of the Environment, Transport and the Regions (1998) *1998 Index of Local Deprivation*, London, DETR.

Field, B. and MacGregor, B. (1987) *Forecasting Techniques for Urban and Regional Planning*, London, Hutchinson.

Foreman, A. (1996) 'Health needs assessment', in Percy-Smith, J. (ed.) *Needs Assessment in Public Policy*, pp. 66–81, Buckingham, Open University Press.

Gephart, R. (1988) *Ethnostatistics: The Qualitative Foundation for Quantitative Research*, Qualitative Research Methods series, No. 12, New York, Sage.

Green, J. and Hart, L. (1999) 'The impact of context on data', in Barbour, R. and Kitzinger, J. (eds) *Developing Focus Group Research: Politics, Theory and Practice*, pp. 21–35, London, Sage.

Holton, S. and Needham, G. (1995) *Successful Purchasing: From Information to Action*, London, King's Fund College.

Jarman, B. (1983) 'Identification of underprivileged areas', *British Medical Journal*, Vol. 286, pp. 1705–59.

Jarman, B., Hirsch, S., White, P. and Driscoll, R. (1992) 'Predicting psychiatric admission rates', *British Medical Journal*, Vol. 304, pp. 1146–51.

Jowell, T., Larrier, C. and Lawrence, R. (1990) *Joint CCSAP/King's Fund Centre Action Project into the Needs of Carers in Black and Minority Communities in Birmingham*, Birmingham, Community Care Special Action Project.

Judge, K. and Mays, N. (1994) 'Allocating resources for health and social care in England', *British Medical Journal*, Vol. 308, pp. 1363–66.

Kind, P., Dolan, P., Gudex, C. and Williams, A. (1998) 'Variations in population health status: results from a United Kingdom national questionnaire survey', *British Medical Journal*, Vol. 316, pp. 736–41.

Kish, L. (1965) *Survey Sampling*, London, John Wiley and Sons.

Krueger, R. (1994) *Focus Groups: A Practical Guide for Applied Research* (2nd edn), London, Sage.

Local Government Management Board (1994) *Information for Caring – GIS in Social Services*, London, LGMB.

McColl, A., Roderick, P., Gabbay, J., Smith, H. and Moore, M. (1998) 'Performance indicators for primary care groups: an evidence-based approach', *British Medical Journal*, Vol. 317, pp. 1354–60.

McConway, K. (ed.) (1994) *Studying Health and Disease*, Buckingham, Open University Press.

McIver, S. (1998) *Healthy Debate? An Independent Evaluation of Citizen Juries in Health Settings*, London, King's Fund Publishing.

Meltzer, D. (1992) *Dementia: Epidemiologically Based Needs Assessment*, Review No. 16, Bristol, Health Care Evaluation Unit, University of Bristol.

Mirrlees-Black, C. (1998) *Rural Areas and Crime: Findings from the British Crime Survey*, Research Findings No. 77, London, Home Office.

Mirrlees-Black, C. and Byron, C. (1998) *Domestic Violence: Findings from the BCS Self-Completion Questionnaire*, Research Findings No. 86, London, Home Office.

National Health Service Executive (1998) *The New NHS, Modern and Dependable: A National Framework for Assessing Performance*, London, Department of Health.

National Health Service Management Executive (1991) *Assessing Health Care Needs*, London, NHSME.

Nazroo, J. (1997a) *Ethnicity and Mental Health: Findings from a Community Survey*, London, Policy Studies Institute.

Nazroo, J. (1997b) *The Health of Britain's Ethnic Minorities*, London, Policy Studies Institute.

Noble, M. and Smith, T. (1994) 'Children in need: using geographical information systems to inform strategic planning for social service provision', *Children and Society*, Vol. 8, No. 4, pp. 360–76.

Payne, N. and Saul, C. (1997) 'Variations in use of cardiology services in a health authority: comparison of coronary artery revascularisation rates with prevalence of angina and coronary mortality', *British Medical Journal*, Vol. 314, pp. 257–66.

Percy-Smith, J. (1996) 'Assessing community needs', in Percy-Smith, J. (ed.) *Needs Assessment in Public Policy*, pp. 82–97, Buckingham, Open University Press.

Porteous, D. (1996) 'Methodologies for needs assessment', in Percy-Smith, J. (ed.) *Needs Assessment in Public Policy*, pp. 32–46, Buckingham, Open University Press.

Sampson, A. and Phillips, C. (1992) *Multiple Victimisation: Racial Attacks on an East London Housing Estate*, Crime Prevention Unit Paper 36, London, Home Office.

Smaje, C. (1995) *Health, 'Race' and Ethnicity: Making Sense of the Evidence*, London, King's Fund Institute/Share.

Stevens, A. and Gillam, S. (1998) 'Needs assessment: from theory to practice', *British Medical Journal*, Vol. 316, pp. 1448–52.

Stevens, A. and Raftery, J. (1994) *Health Care Needs Assessment: The Epidemiological-Based Needs Assessment Reviews*, Oxford, Radcliffe Medical Press.

Stevens, A. and Raftery, J. (1997) *Health Care Needs Assessment: The Epidemiological-Based Needs Assessment Reviews Second Series*, Oxford, Radcliffe Medical Press.

Townsend, P., Simpson, P. and Tibbs, N. (1985) 'Inequalities in health in the city of Bristol: a preliminary review of the statistical evidence', *International Journal of Health Services*, Vol. 15, pp. 637–43.

Townsend, P., Phillimore, P. and Beattie, A. (1988) *Health and Deprivation: Inequality in the North*, Beckenham, Croom Helm.

Unwin, N., Carr, S., Leeson, J. and Pless-Mulloli, T. (1997) *An Introductory Guide to Public Health and Epidemiology*, Buckingham, Open University Press.

White, K., Williams, T. and Greenberg, B. (1961) 'The ecology of medical care', *New England Journal of Medicine*, Vol. 265, pp. 885–92.

Williams, R. and Wright, J. (1998) 'Epidemiological issues in health needs assessment', *British Medical Journal*, Vol. 316, pp. 1379–82.

Appendix: Accessing evidence – an overview of sources of information for evidence-based practice

Introduction

The range of information sources available to practitioners to support evidence-based practice is growing at a bewildering rate. A major UK-wide initiative – the National Electronic Library for Health – should revolutionise access to health information for both practitioners and the public. Similar plans are under way in social care, beginning with free access to the National Institute for Social Work's *Caredata* database throughout Scotland, funded by the Scottish Executive. These initiatives will, ultimately, offer the distinct advantage of a single initial access-point to information. Meanwhile, however, the rate of change means that it would be futile to attempt to produce an exhaustive directory of recommended information sources – any such directory would be out of date well before publication. It is also recognised that access to computers is by no means universal, although it is increasing all the time. This appendix, therefore, merely provides a series of signposts to information sources for evidence-based practice, and strongly suggests that the reader uses the recommended Internet sources, or contacts the specialist organisations, to identify the most up-to-date solutions and initiatives.

While no attempt is made here to cover techniques of accessing information, they are discussed in the companion volume to this one: Gomm, R., Needham, G. and Bullman, A. (eds) (2000) *Evaluating Research in Health and Social Care*, London, Sage in association with The Open University (K302 Reader 2).

1   Printed sources – books, journals and reports

Books

This is a small selection from the many evidence-based practice textbooks.

Evidence-based Healthcare: How to Make Health Policy and Management Decisions

Gray, J. A. M. (1997) Churchill Livingstone, ISBN 0-443-05721-4.

A practical guide for people who manage or purchase health services or make health policies, condensed from the practical experiences of many people and projects.

Evidence Based Healthcare: A Practical Guide for Therapists

Bury, T. J. and Mead, J. M. (1998) Butterworth-Heinemann,
ISBN 0-750-63783-8.

Evidence-based Medicine: How to Practice and Teach EBM

Sackett, D. L. *et al.* (1997) Churchill Livingstone, ISBN 0-443-05686-2.

An explanation of how to apply the key principles of evidence-based
practice in your everyday clinical work.

Evidence-based Social Work Practice with Families: A Lifespan Approach

Corcoran, J. (2000) Springer, ISBN 0-826-11303-6.

How to Read a Paper: The Basics of Evidence Based Medicine

Greenhalgh, T. (1997) BMJ Publishing Group, ISBN 0-7279-1139-2.

This book aims to introduce non-experts to finding medical articles and
assessing their value. It has also been published as a 'How to read a paper'
series in the *British Medical Journal*.

The ScHARR Guide to Evidence-based Practice (1997)

A bibliography and resource guide produced by:

ScHARR Information Resources
University of Sheffield
Regent Court
30 Regent Street
Sheffield S1 4DA.

This guide can be downloaded from the main ScHARR 'Netting the
Evidence' Web site and is freely distributed within the university and NHS
sectors.

Web site: **http://www.shef.ac.uk/~scharr/ir/ebpfin.doc**

Journals and newsletters

While relevant research articles may be found in the majority of
professional and academic journals in health and social care, there are
also journals specialising in reviewing the results of research and its
relevance for practice. These include the following.

Bandolier

NHS monthly newsletter on local and national initiatives and literature on
the effectiveness of health care interventions.

Clinical Effectiveness in Nursing

Quarterly nursing journal focusing on the effectiveness of clinical interventions.

Clinical Evidence

Six-monthly, updated compendium of evidence on the effects of common clinical interventions from the BMJ Publishing Group.

Effective Health Care Bulletins

Bi-monthly bulletin from the Centre for Reviews and Dissemination which examines the effectiveness of a variety of health care interventions, summarises results and makes clear recommendations for practice. Distributed free within the NHS.

Effectiveness Matters

Annual updates on the effectiveness of important health interventions for practitioners and decision-makers in the NHS. Distributed free within the NHS.

Evidence-Based Health Care

Bi-monthly journal that aims to provide managers with the best evidence available about the financing, organisation and delivery of health care.

Evidence-Based Medicine

Bi-monthly journal that alerts clinicians to important advances in all areas of medicine. It is also available as CD-ROM 'Best Evidence'.

Evidence-Based Mental Health

Quarterly journal containing clinically useful and accurate selected articles on clinically relevant advances in treatment and the organisation of care, diagnosis, aetiology, prognosis/outcome research, quality improvement, continuing education, and economic evaluation.

Evidence-Based Nursing

Quarterly journal that identifies and appraises high quality, clinically relevant research.

Evidence-Based Social Care Newsletter

Published three times a year by the Centre for Evidence-Based Social Services (CEBSS).

Health Evidence Bulletins, Wales

Signposts to the best current evidence across a broad range of evidence types and subject areas.

Health Expectations

Quarterly journal aiming to promote critical thinking and informed debate about all aspects of public participation in health care and health policy.

Journal of Clinical Effectiveness

Quarterly journal focusing on evidence-based practice, clinical effectiveness, guidelines and clinical audit.

Journal of Evaluation in Clinical Practice

Quarterly journal containing articles and systematic reviews of research on clinical effectiveness and the implementation of evidence-based care.

Journal of Health and Social Policy

Covers many health and health-related professions and focuses on all aspects of policy – its development, formulation, implementation, evaluation, review and revision.

Journal of Social Service Research

Exclusively devoted to empirical research and its application to the design, delivery and management of the new social services.

Reports

Reports may provide in-depth coverage of a piece of primary research or an overview and review of several primary research studies. In fields that have many relevant research studies, they can provide an invaluable way of assessing the literature. They may be published by government departments, professional bodies or voluntary organisations. The following are some examples.

CRD (NHS Centre for Reviews and Dissemination) Reports

Discuss the results of a systematic review of research in more depth than an *Effective Health Care Bulletin*. Press releases, executive summaries and some reports in full text are available on their Web site:

http://www.york.ac.uk/inst/crd/crdrep.htm

Department of Health Reports

The Department of Health produces many reports that review the research evidence. These publications may be traced using the POINT search engine available at:

http://www.doh.gov.uk/pointh.htm

Details are also available from the Health Literature line: tel. 0800 555 777.

Reports may be published as White and Green Papers, but often as other Department of Health series: for example, the guidance on commissioning cancer series, which summarise the research evidence on questions about improving outcomes for cancer treatments, or the Confidential Enquiry reports into areas such as maternal and infant deaths.

Development and Evaluation Committee Reports

The Development and Evaluation service aims to provide commissioners in South West and South East England with reliable, timely information about the cost-effectiveness of health care technologies. The reports contain information on the quality of evidence for both proposed and current treatments, and a measure of effect size and costs.

Web site: **http://www.hta.nhsweb.nhs.uk/rapidhta**

Health Technology Assessment Reports

Results of the NHS Health Technology Assessment Programme into the costs, effectiveness and broader impacts of health technologies are published as reports, many available in full text.

Web site: **http://www.hta.nhsweb.nhs.uk**

Joseph Rowntree Foundation Reports

This organisation's programme of R&D projects in housing, social care and social policy are published in various formats. Details are available on their Web site:

http://www.jrf.org.uk

University of York Social Policy Research Unit Reports

The Unit produces a series of publications including SPRU papers (short reports providing up-to-the-minute commentary as well as a reflective and critical presentation of research and research findings) and Social Policy Reports (covering research findings, comments on methodology, and discussion of policy and practice).

Web site: **http://www.york.ac.uk/inst/spru**

2 Electronic sources – on-line databases and Internet resources

Databases

The following selection of databases can be used to search for evidence-based practice information. Some or all of them should be available in specialist health care/social care or academic libraries.

AgeInfo

A CD-ROM database on age and ageing from the Centre for Policy on Ageing.

AMED (Allied and Alternative Medicine)

Offers access to resources in non-traditional medicine and covers reference articles from 350 journals, many not indexed elsewhere.

Best Evidence

A CD-ROM database of abstracts from ACP Journal Club (since 1991) and Evidence-Based Medicine (since 1995) which covers reviews from more than 90 journals world-wide.

British Nursing Index (BNI)

A database of articles from over 220 nursing journals, available in printed form, on CD-ROM and on the Internet.

CANCERLIT

Covers the treatment of cancer and information on epidemiology, pathogenesis and immunology.

Caredata

Contains abstracts of books, research papers and journal articles from social work and social care publications and is available on CD-ROM and the Internet.

CINAHL (Cumulative Index to Nursing and Allied Health Literature)

This database covers all aspects of nursing and allied health disciplines such as health education, occupational therapy, emergency services and social services in health care.

Cochrane Library

This is the premier source of information on the effectiveness of health care interventions. It is produced by the Cochrane Collaboration, an international network of people committed to 'preparing, maintaining, and disseminating systematic, up-to-date reviews of the effects of health care'. It contains the following databases.

Cochrane Database of Systematic Reviews (CDSR)

A rapidly growing collection of regularly updated, systematic reviews of the effects of health care.

Database of Abstracts of Reviews of Effectiveness (DARE)

Includes structured abstracts of systematic reviews from around the world. Also available through the CRD (NHS Centre for Reviews and Dissemination – see under 'Reports').

Cochrane Controlled Trials Register (CCTR)

A bibliography of controlled trials as part of an international effort to hand-search the world's journals and create an unbiased source of data for systematic reviews.

Cochrane Review Methodology Database (CRMD)

A bibliography of articles on the science of research synthesis and on practical aspects of preparing systematic reviews.

ACP Journal Club Abstracts

Available on CD-ROM and the Internet.

EMBASE

The European equivalent of MEDLINE (see entry below), the Excerpta Medica database focuses on drugs and pharmacology. Other aspects of human medicine covered include health policy, drug and alcohol dependence, psychiatry, forensic science and pollution control.

ENB Health Care Database

References and abstracts from more than 80 UK journals, since 1985, produced by the English National Board (ENB) for Nursing, Midwifery and Health Visiting.

Web site: **http://www.enb.org.uk/hcd.htm**

Health-CD

A database launched in 1997 of many publications and documents from the Department of Health and the Stationery Office.

HealthSTAR

Covers literature on the non-clinical aspects of health care delivery such as administration and planning of health care facilities and evaluation of patient outcomes. It is available on CD-ROM, on the Internet or on hard disk and is international (published in the USA).

Health Technology Assessment (HTA) Database

Contains abstracts produced by INAHTA (International Network of Agencies for Health Technology Assessment) and other health care technology agencies.

HMIC (Health Management Information Consortium)

This database consists of the combined catalogues of the Department of Health, the King's Fund and the Nuffield Institute for Health, whose main subject focus is health care management in the UK. It is available on CD-ROM.

MEDLINE

The US National Library of Medicine's bibliographic database covering all aspects of medicine and health care since 1985.

National Research Register (NRR)

Contains 42,000 project records recording ongoing research primarily funded by the NHS.

NHS Economic Evaluation Database (NEED)

This database is produced by the CRD and contains abstracts of economic evaluations of health technologies (since 1990).

Outcomes Activities Database

Contains details of recently completed activities connected with health outcomes work in all settings within the health service.

PsycLIT/PsycInfo

Contains abstracts of the world's journal literature in psychology and related disciplines and is compiled from the PsycInfo database. It is available on CD-ROM.

SIGLE (System for Information on Grey Literature in Europe)

Grey literature is best defined as literature that is difficult to identify or obtain. This database is available on CD-ROM or hard disk.

Internet resources

The Internet is an excellent resource for evidence-based practice information. Several sites act as gateways to the huge range of information available.

Core List for Evidence-Based Practice

A list of books, reports and journals suggested as a starting point for a UK library or clinical audit/effectiveness unit.

Web site:
http://www.shef.ac.uk/uni/academic/R-Z/scharr/ir/corelist.html

CTI [Computers in Teaching Initiative] Centre for Human Services – Social Work

A gateway to sites with information on education, research and training for social work teaching and practice.

Web site: **http://www.soton.ac.uk/~chst**

Drs.Desk

The Doctors Desk is an integrated desk-top information and communications system that a GP needs for evidence-based practice.

Web site: **http://drsdesk.sghms.ac.uk**

Evidence-based health electronic discussion list

For teachers and practitioners in health-related fields; to announce meetings and courses; stimulate discussion; air controversies; and aid the implementation of evidence-based health. To subscribe:

E-mail: mailbase@mailbase.ac.uk

Other discussion lists of interest can be browsed through, and subscribed to, via the Mailbase Web site at the University of Newcastle:
http://www.ncl.ac.uk/ucs/email/mailbase.html

Evidence Based Health Care – A Resource Pack

Reading and key references concerning the background and current thinking on evidence-based health care and details of the groups and organisations involved in this movement.

Web site: **http://drsdesk.sghms.ac.uk/Starnet/pack.htm**

McMaster University EBM

A Canadian site containing a huge amount of evidence-based health care information and links to other useful resources.

Web site: **http://www-hsl.mcmaster.ca/ebm**

Nursing and Health Care Resources on the Net

Helps you find the Internet source that most closely meets your interest.

Web site: **http://www.shef.ac.uk/~nhcon**

OMNI (Organising Medical Networked Information)

A gateway to Internet resources in medicine, biomedicine, allied health, health management and related topics.

Web site: **http://omni.ac.uk**

ScHARR (Sheffield School of Health and Related Research) – Lock's Guide to the Evidence

A guide to printed sources of evidence, focusing on grey literature from UK academic and quasi-governmental sources.

Web site:
http://www.shef.ac.uk/uni/academic/R-Z/scharr/ir/scebm.html

ScHARR (Sheffield School of Health and Related Research) – Netting the Evidence

An on-line guide to journal articles, contact organisations, Internet discussion groups and definitions in all areas of evidence-based practice.

E-mail: a.booth@sheffield.ac.uk

Web site: **http://www.shef.ac.uk/~scharr/ir/netting.html**

SOSIG (Social Science Information Gateway)

Internet resources gateway covering sociology, psychology and social welfare.

Web site: **http://www.sosig.ac.uk/**

3   Projects, initiatives and organisations

Aggressive Research Intelligence Facility (ARIF)

A specialist unit at the University of Birmingham set up to help health care workers access and interpret research evidence in response to particular problems.

Telephone/fax/answering system: 0121 414 7878

Web site: **http://www.hsrc.org.uk/links/arif/arifhome.htm**

Centre for Evidence-Based Child Health

Aims to increase the provision of effective and efficient child health care through an educational programme for health professionals.

Telephone: +44 (0) 171 905 2606

Fax: +44 (0) 171 813 8233

E-mail: rgilbert@ich.ucl.ac.uk

Web site: **http://www.ich.bpmf.ac.uk/ebm/ebm.htm**

Centre for Evidence-Based Medicine

Aims to promote evidence-based health care and provide support and resources to anyone working or interested in the field. The CEBM Web site has links to other bodies and organisations.

Telephone: 01865 221321

Web site: **http://cebm.jr2.ox.ac.uk**

Centre for Evidence-Based Mental Health

Provides resources for promoting and supporting the teaching and practice of evidence-based mental health care, including the journal *Evidence-Based Mental Health*, the Royal College of Psychiatrists' guidelines in full-text, and OXAMWEB (a mental health evidence links site).

Telephone: +44 (0) 1865 226476

Fax: +44 (0) 1865 793101

E-mail: cebmh.enquiries@psychiatry.ox.ac.uk

Web site: **http://www.psychiatry.ox.ac.uk/cebmh**

Centre for Evidence-Based Nursing

Identifies evidence-based practice through primary research and systematic reviews and promotes the uptake of evidence into practice through education and implementation activities.

Telephone: 01904 435222/435137

Fax: 01904 435225

E-mail: health.matters@pulse.york.ac.uk

Web site:
http://www.york.ac.uk/depts/hstd/centres/evidence/ev-intro.htm

Centre for Evidence-Based Pharmacotherapy (CEBP)

Researches the methodology of medicines assessment, pharmaco-epidemiology and pharmacoeconomics.

Aston University
Aston Triangle
Birmingham B4 7ET

Telephone: +44 (0) 121 359 3611

Web site: **http://www.aston.ac.uk/pharmacy/cebp**

Centre for Evidence-Based Social Services (CEBSS)

Aims to improve the knowledge base of social work education and practice and to facilitate the implementation of research findings.

University of Exeter
Amory Building
Rennes Drive
Exeter EX4 4RJ

Telephone: 01392 263323

E-mail: S.E.Bosley@exeter.ac.uk

Web site: **http://www.ex.ac.uk/cebss**

Centre for Health Information Quality

Supports the development of patient information that is clearly communicated, evidence-based and involves patients.

Telephone: 01962 863511 ext. 200

Fax: 01962 849079

E-mail: enquiries@centreforhiq.demon.co.uk

CRD (NHS Centre for Reviews and Dissemination)

Funded by the NHS as part of its Research and Development Strategy, the CRD aims to review the effectiveness of health care interventions and to disseminate the findings to key decision-makers in the NHS and to consumers of health care services.

General enquiries: telephone 01904 433634

Information service: telephone 01904 433707

Web site: **http://www.york.ac.uk/inst/crd/welcome.htm**

Dynamic Quality Improvement Network (DQI Network)

Part of the Royal College of Nursing's DQI Programme which includes a range of activities relating to clinical effectiveness, clinical guidelines, clinical audit and quality improvement.

Web site: **http://www.rcn.org.uk/services/promote/quality/quality.htm#dqi**

FACTS (Framework for Appropriate Care Throughout Sheffield) Project

A project developing methods to help GPs tackle effectiveness in their practice.

Telephone: 0114 275 5658

E-mail: Facts@Sheffield.ac.uk

Web site: **http://www.shef.ac.uk/uni/projects/facts**

King's Fund Library

An independent health policy organisation, the King's Fund Library is concerned with health care management and organisational development and has a range of 'grey literature'.

Telephone: +44 (0) 20 7307 2568/9

Fax: +44 (0) 20 7307 2805

Web site: **http://www.Kingsfund.org.uk/eLibrary/html/library_main.htm**

MIDIRS (Midwives Information and Resource Service)

A charity providing information to health professionals involved in maternity care through a variety of sources.

Telephone: 0800 581009

E-mail: midirs@dial.pipex.com

Web site: **http://www.midirs.org**

National Centre for Clinical Audit (NCCA)

Aims to improve the quality of clinical audit activities within the NHS. Also holds databases. The Web site and functions of this Centre are being absorbed and incorporated into the National Institute for Clinical Excellence (NICE – see entry overleaf).

National Co-ordinating Centre for Health Technology Assessment (NCCHTA)

Funded by the Department of Health, this initiative between the Wessex Institute for Health Research and Development at Southampton University and the University of York aims to support and develop the NHS Health Technology Assessment programme.

Centre for Health Economics
University of York
York YO10 5DD

Telephone: 01904 433718

E-mail: CHEweb@york.ac.uk

Web site: **http://www.york.ac.uk/inst/che/2314.htm**

National Electronic Library for Health (NELH)

The aims of the NELH are to provide easy access to best current knowledge and to improve health and health care, clinical practice and patient choice. Details of the developing Library and its Virtual Branch Libraries are on the Web site:

http://www.nelh.nhs.uk/

or can be obtained from:

Robert Ward
NHS Information Authority
Room 1 N35C Quarry House
Quarry Hill
Leeds LS2 7UE

Telephone: 0113 254 6245

E-mail: robward@doh.gov.uk

National Institute for Clinical Excellence (NICE)

A national NHS initiative launched in April 1999. The Institute was set up to appraise health interventions and will offer clinicians and managers guidance on the best treatments for patients. It will act as a centre of guidance for health professionals in the NHS, as well as patients and the general public. The Institute has also absorbed the functions of the National Centre for Clinical Audit (NCCA) – see entry above.

NICE
90 Long Acre
Covent Garden
London WC2E 9RZ

Telephone: 0171 849 3444

Fax: 0171 849 3162

E-mail: ncca@ncca.org.uk

Web site: **http://www.nice.org.uk**

National Institute for Social Work (NISW)

NISW is one of the groups looking after professionals working in the social care and social welfare fields. It provides professional development opportunities and information for both practitioners and users of social care services in the UK. It is involved with the latest initiatives to set up a new National Electronic Library for Social Care, and produces the *Caredata Abstracts* database, now available free to people in Scotland.

Web site: **http://www.nisw.org.uk**

National Primary Care Research and Development Centre (NPCRDC)

A multidisciplinary centre aiming to improve primary and community health care in the NHS through the generation, dissemination and application of knowledge and ideas relevant to the funding, organisation and delivery of health services.

Telephone: 0161 275 7633

Fax: 0161 275 7600

E-mail: maria.cairney@man.ac.uk

Web site: **http://www.cpcr.man.ac.uk**

UK Cochrane Centre

The UK headquarters of the international Cochrane Collaboration. Aims to facilitate, maintain and disseminate systematic, up-to-date reviews of randomised controlled trials of health care.

Telephone: +44 (0) 1865 516300

Fax: +44 (0) 1865 516311

E-mail: general@cochrane.co.uk

Web site: **http://www.update-software.com/ccweb/default.html**

WISDOM Project

A pilot project to create an on-line environment, using the Internet to train primary care professionals in informatics, evidence-based practice being a focus of the group.

WISDOM Centre
Institute of General Practice and Primary Care
Community Sciences Centre
Northern General Hospital
Sheffield S5 7AU

Telephone: 0114 271 5095

E-mail: n.j.fox@Sheffield.ac.uk

Web site: **http://www.shef.ac.uk/uni/projects/wrp/index.html**

Index

4, 5 Dec
29, 30 Jan
26, 27 Mar
21, 22 May
9, 10 Jul